The Diffusion and Va[lue of]
HEALTHCARE
Information Technology

Anthony G. Bower

Sponsored by Cerner Corporation, General Electric, Hewlett-Packard, Johnson & Johnson, and Xerox

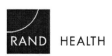

RAND HEALTH

The research described in this report was conducted within RAND Health and sponsored by a consortium of private companies, including Cerner Corporation, General Electric, Hewlett-Packard, Johnson & Johnson, and Xerox.

Library of Congress Cataloging-in-Publication Data

Bower, Anthony G.
  The diffusion and value of healthcare information technology / Anthony G. Bower.
    p. cm.
    "MG-272."
    Includes bibliographical references.
    ISBN 0-8330-3760-9 (pbk. : alk. paper)
    1. Medicine—Information technology—Evaluation. 2. Medicine—Information technology—Government policy—United States. 3. Medical records—Data processing—Cost effectiveness. 4. Diffusion of innovations.
    [DNLM: 1. Diffusion of innovation. 2. Medical Records Systems, Computerized—utilization. 3. Information Systems.] I. Title.

R858.B68 2005
610'.28—dc22

                                                                    2005002944

The RAND Corporation is a nonprofit research organization providing objective analysis and effective solutions that address the challenges facing the public and private sectors around the world. RAND's publications do not necessarily reflect the opinions of its research clients and sponsors.

RAND® is a registered trademark.

A profile of RAND Health, abstracts of its publications, and ordering information can be found on the RAND Health home page at www.rand.org/health.

Cover design by Barbara Angell Caslon

© Copyright 2005 RAND Corporation

Published 2005 by the RAND Corporation
1776 Main Street, P.O. Box 2138, Santa Monica, CA 90407-2138
1200 South Hayes Street, Arlington, VA 22202-5050
201 North Craig Street, Suite 202, Pittsburgh, PA 15213-1516
RAND URL: http://www.rand.org/
To order RAND documents or to obtain additional information, contact
Distribution Services: Telephone: (310) 451-7002;
Fax: (310) 451-6915; Email: order@rand.org

Preface

This report presents research on the diffusion and value of healthcare information technology (HIT). It is part of a larger RAND Corporation study that examined the value of HIT and policy options available to promote HIT, if and when such promotion seems appropriate. Future reports from the larger study are anticipated to be published in the middle of 2005.

Healthcare faces multiple problems, including high and rising expenditures, inconsistent quality, and gaps in care and access. Healthcare information technology, and especially complex electronic health records (EHRs), have been thought to be possible partial solutions to those problems.

This report characterizes the diffusion of electronic health records and places that diffusion within a theoretical diffusion framework. EHR diffusion, once the theory is understood, is for the most part intuitive and explainable. The report then answers the question of how much healthcare information technology might be worth to society. It analyzes other industries to arrive at a theory of information technology (IT) value and then creates plausible healthcare scenarios and quantifies the benefits.

Finally, the report analyzes potential IT market failures in healthcare and identifies some possible policy directions.

This research was conducted within RAND Health, a division of the RAND Corporation. It was sponsored by a generous consortium of private companies, including Cerner, General Electric, Hewlett Packard, Johnson & Johnson, and Xerox. The right to publish any results was retained by RAND.

The report should be of interest to information technology professionals, healthcare executives, and government officials responsible for health policy.

Contents

Figures

Tables

Summary

Virtually no one would argue that the $1.6 trillion spent annually (as of 2002) on U.S. healthcare is spent efficiently. Americans are not any healthier than citizens in most other developed nations, despite the mammoth expenditures.

There is a well-documented productivity renaissance in the U.S. economy, dating from the mid-1990s. A number of prominent industries, including wholesaling and retailing, have greatly increased productivity over the last decade.[1] At the heart of their efforts was information technology (IT) transformation, although not all heavy IT-using industries have experienced increased productivity.

The purpose of this study is to investigate four sets of questions designed to help determine if healthcare can duplicate the IT-enabled gains seen in other industries, and if so, how:

- What is the current diffusion of HIT, especially the complex electronic health record (EHR) systems[2] that hold out the promise of healthcare transformation?
- How does EHR diffusion compare to other innovations, especially IT innovations, in other industries? And how fast will EHR likely diffuse if the healthcare system does nothing differently?
- How much would HIT diffusion likely be worth to society (1) if nothing is done differently and also (2) if adoption were quickened?
- What should the government do, if anything, to assist in the purchase or implementation of HIT and specifically EHR? Is speeding the adoption of EHR worth the costs of doing so?

---

[1] The primary productivity measure used in this report is labor productivity, which is simply output divided by labor hours.

[2] A basic EHR system provides electronic remote user access of results in the form of text, including lab reports, radiology, transcribed notes, current medications, problems, demographics, and possibly some scanned reports. More advanced EHR systems have guideline-based content and patient- and condition-specific reminders, population management, and interprovider communication.

Brief Overview of Research Approach

To answer the question of the current diffusion of HIT (Chapter Two), we analyzed an industry data source and compared our results to others' results. To answer the question of why HIT has diffused the way that it has (Chapter Three), we surveyed the diffusion literature to find diffusion drivers and then assessed HIT and particularly EHR on those drivers.

Part of our assessment relied on a series of surveys and interviews conducted at facilities that were using or contemplating the use of EHR. Our survey used a purposive sample of a variety of healthcare stakeholders identified through literature and expert recommendations. Sixteen sites were visited. Later visits were specifically to gather cost and HIT-related process improvement information from sites identified as engaging in these activities.

Site visits were supported by telephone interviews with leading HIT professionals. The site visit goals included fact finding and hypothesis development, identifying barriers, enablers, value measurement, range of implementation strategies, and costs.

The second part of our assessment relied on an extensive literature review. The two approaches when combined yielded a prediction of future EHR diffusion. To answer the question of what HIT (and especially EHR) diffusion is worth to the nation (Chapter Four), we found case studies that identified the worth of IT in other industries. We synthesized the case studies and other literature to arrive at a cross-industry theory of IT value and assessed HIT on those drivers using information from literature and interviews with providers. Finally, in asking the question of how or why should government help (Chapter Five), we started from a welfare economics perspective and attempted to identify failures in the HIT market, if any. Our review of all of the evidence from our interviews and the HIT implementation and policy literature revealed several market failures, and on that basis we recommend further study of specific plausible policy interventions.

Our key findings are summarized below.

- EHR is diffusing at a rate consistent with other similar IT technologies in other industries. EHR diffusion is explicable using modern diffusion theory applicable to complex, highly networked IT products.
- Complex electronic medical records are, after a 20-year waiting period, rapidly diffusing in many segments of our healthcare system, with about 30 percent of acute-care hospital providers reporting by the end of 2003 that they had ordered EHR products, and will reach 80 percent saturation in hospitals by about 2016—or earlier if assisted by government or other organizations. Diffusion among physicians' offices is 10–16 percent, depending on the measure.
- More important than hastening adoption, which appears to have taken off since 1999 without intervention, is ensuring that appropriate incentives are in place so that complex EHRs will be used effectively.

- The benefits of the current increase in HIT spending are arguably a *cumulative* 1 percent per year,[3] but the range varies widely depending on what else the government and healthcare players do. Other industries have shown quantifiable IT labor productivity benefits ranging from 0 percent to perhaps 4 percent per year.
- Speeding up adoption may be beneficial, although it depends on the presence of other factors such as competition and regulation. There is very strong evidence that HIT will complement other pro-productivity features such as competition and deregulation. HIT is an enabler of change in how work gets accomplished. This is especially true of complex electronic medical records.

Promising Policy Avenues Identified by This Research

Our research has revealed a number of attractive policy avenues that deserve further study. The policy avenues discussed below are active priorities among the many policymaking stakeholders. The purpose of this report has been to provide a better conceptual and empirical basis for pursuing certain general lines of policy, rather than to discuss specific current proposals in much depth (which are better addressed in a series of ongoing, brief issue papers, for example, than in full reports). Note also that the list below is still very broad. The question may be asked: Ultimately, is HIT not a narrower concern within healthcare, albeit an important one, that deserves a shorter and less ambitious list? There are at least two reasons for the broad list below. First, HIT and especially EHR is a technology that affects virtually all players in the healthcare community. It is a broad technology and requires broad policy to be effective.

Second, the value of HIT is maximized when complementary investments are made. The value of HIT swings widely (perhaps by a factor of 10) depending on what else is going on in the system. In healthcare, there is a lot going on, much of it unhelpful to maximizing the HIT investment. Accordingly, the policy remit to optimize HIT efficiency touches on a number of healthcare problems, many all too familiar to health policymakers.

This report's research lends support to developing policy and solutions in the following broad policy avenues:

Coordinate standards immediately. It is important to continue to coordinate standards and push for initiatives that improve the chances for interoperability, especially within regional communities. Standards should be improved without reducing competition among competing EHR vendors.

---

[3] That is, benefits in the first year are a 1 percent increase in labor productivity, in the second year a 2 percent increase, in the third year a 3 percent increase, and so on, for as long as IT continues to change the organization of work within an industry.

Work to improve quality measurement. The benefits of improving quality measurement are twofold: First, improving quality measurement will help to overcome the healthcare market failure of inadequately recognizing quality, which will spur the adoption of quality-improving innovation, including EHR. Second, there is a feedback loop: Adoption itself will reduce this market failure, because EHR holds the promise of improving quality measurement, largely by automating an otherwise dauntingly labor-intensive process of quality management. This difficulty in measuring and competing on quality is arguably the most important problem in healthcare and EHR could be an important part of the solution.

In addition to these two strong rationales for policy in this area, there is still a third: The government is not just a regulator but a key customer and has the opportunity and indeed the right to improve provider cost effectiveness over time. A strong series of results in the theory of innovation show that a "smart buyer" can drive an industry to higher efficiency. (For example, consider the effects of Japanese consumers' tastes in consumer electronics on Japanese consumer electronics companies.) To date, the government as a buyer has done much to affect the system but much less to reform the system. HIT can help transform the system and help government push through complementary changes in quality measurement and pay for performance that should improve the system. Perhaps this is the area that holds out the greatest promise for truly transformative change.

Reduce network externalities.[4] The government can work to lessen network externalities, which should lead to more adoption of EHR and especially more effective adoption. Our analysis suggests that the federal government could lead an intervention, but a successful policy needs to encourage linking the local providers for any specific patient. To assist with these efforts, the government may need to consider further relaxing inurement of benefit regulations with respect to HIT. Because of network externalities, some selective grants or subsidies *may* be optimal for underfunded physicians' offices, but we do not view this as proven. Alternatively, allowing transfer payments (connect fees or bonuses) among members of the regional network may be a good idea (and less expensive for the government). The allowed financial incentives should be targeted at improving community connectivity directly (e.g., IT hardware), or indirectly (e.g., digitizing patient paper records). However, there needs to be further, detailed research at the firm and regional level to guide policy here.

Recognize that HIT requires complementary investments. It has been shown in other industries that IT is much more effective when combined with vigorous competition and deregulation. Complex IT such as EHR is definitely not a standalone or plug-and-play type of benefit. Rather, it can, if (and only if) used appropri-

---

[4] A network externality exists when a user's benefit *increases* as the number of other users increases. A fax machine is an example of an IT innovation with network externalities.

ately, deliver dramatic changes in the overall delivery of care that could radically improve quality and lower the cost of delivering that higher quality.

The reverse side of this observation is that preventing complementary changes in work processes by stifling competition or direct regulation might prevent HIT gains from occurring.

Make policy decisions that turn HIT into a competitive weapon. Industrial history shows that IT is most efficiently used when used as a competitive weapon central to a firm's business. This result is highly consistent with a more general theory of successful innovation in a modern economy. In the context of health policy, one way to sharpen the competitive advantage of IT might be to reimburse quality in Medicare more directly, where measuring quality is possible only with an EHR-enabled quality tracking system. Another fruitful line of research would be to study whether Medicare should pay for EHR-enabled claims. In such a world, providers improve profitability by using EHR and using it well and having the credible quality measures to prove that they are using it well. (Note that this policy prescription is related to the quality-measurement policies above, because they both address the fundamental market failure of poorly measured quality.)

Discuss and agree whether 100 percent EHR penetration is a societal goal, because history suggests that it will not happen without intervention. EHR diffusion has reached more than 20 percent of acute-care hospitals and may soon go over 50 percent. However, the analysis in Chapter Two suggests, based on review of other IT innovations, that penetration will not reach 100 percent of the provider community. If 100 percent EHR is a societal goal, because society wishes to maximize network gains or avoid a two-tier system, or both, then some form of subsidy for the more disadvantaged and isolated practices is likely necessary. The issues for these offices should likely be interoperability and community connectivity to maximize gains from HIT and EHR in particular.

Adopt an incremental, evolutionary perspective on policy development. There are few more important areas for proper government economic policy than healthcare, specifically HIT. It is only a slight overstatement to say that future U.S. competitiveness and the health of its citizens depend upon it.

Given the enormous stakes, the uncertainty in the effects of policy, and the latency of the gains from HIT implementation, it might be wise to heed organizational theorists' views on evolutionary policy analysis. It is usually best to be able to evaluate policies and business strategies early and adapt quickly. Such a perspective is almost certainly wise in this context.

This suggests incremental government interventions with rapid review of results, with follow-on funding for successful interventions.

Acknowledgments

I wish to thank my colleagues on the project team for their expertise and insights. The research has also benefited from comments from a steering committee, chaired by David Lawrence. A special thanks goes to those who provided detailed comments on drafts, including James Bigelow, Tora Bikson, Robin Meili, Richard Scoville, Roger Taylor, Mary Vaiana, and the project leader, Richard Hillestad, and the two formal reviewers, Emmett Keeler and James Teng.

I also wish to thank Kateryna Fonkych, RAND Graduate School student, for her careful research assistance and for her comments on earlier versions of this report.

Finally, I am most grateful to our research sponsors for their support. They include Cerner, GE, Hewlett Packard, Johnson & Johnson, and Xerox.

Acronyms

4GL	Fourth Generation Language
ACH	Automated Clearing House
AHA	American Hospital Association
ATM	Automated Teller Machine
CAD/CAM	Computer-Assisted Drawing/Computer-Aided Manufacturing
CAGR	Compounded Annual Growth Rate
CASE	Computer Assisted Software Engineering
CDR	Computerized Data Record
CEO	Chief Executive Officer
CIO	Chief Information Officer
CMS	Centers for Medicare and Medicaid Services
CPOE	Computerized Physician Order Entry
CPR	Computerized Patient Records
EDI	Electronic Data Interchange
EHR	Electronic Health Records
EIS	Expanded Inband Signaling
EMR-S	Electronic Medical Record Systems
ERP	Enterprise Resource Planning
GDP	Gross Domestic Product
GM	General Motors
GMS	General Merchandising Services
HIT	Healthcare Information Technology
HMO	Health Maintenance Organization
ICD	International Classification of Diseases

IHDS	Integrated Healthcare Delivery System
ISDN	Integrated Services Data Network
IT	Information Technology
LAN	Local Area Network
LSRD	Large Scale Relational Database
MGI	McKinsey Global Institute
NCVHS	National Committee on Vital and Health Statistics
PACS	Picture Archiving and Communication System
PC	Personal Computer
PITAC	President's Information Technology Advisory Committee
QALY	Quality Adjusted Life Years
RHIO	Regional Heal Initiative Organization
VCR	Video Camera Recorder

CHAPTER ONE

Introduction

Why Is Healthcare Information Technology Diffusion and Its Value Important?

In 2002, the United States spent approximately 15 percent of its gross domestic product (GDP) on healthcare (National Health Expenditure Statistics, 2004). This spending represents the highest proportion in the world and the largest single sector of the U.S. economy. And yet, virtually no one would argue that it is spent efficiently. Americans are not much healthier than citizens in other nations, despite the mammoth expenditures.

There is a well-documented productivity renaissance in the U.S. economy, dating from the mid-1990s (see Nordhaus, 2002, for example). A number of prominent industries, including wholesaling and retailing, have greatly increased productivity over the last decade.[1] At the heart of their efforts was information technology (IT) transformation, although not all heavy IT-using industries have experienced increased productivity. Healthcare IT introduction appears to continue at a relatively rapid pace, but very little evidence to date points to significant productivity improvements in the massive healthcare sector.[2]

At the same time, IT usage in healthcare lags some other industries. HIT expenditures have not accelerated in the last six years, instead only keeping pace with overall healthcare expenditures (see Sheldon Dorenfest and Associates, 2004). A fragmented healthcare system, go-it-alone culture, and seemingly inadequate investment funds (despite the high overall expenditures on healthcare) have appeared to

---

[1] The primary productivity measure is labor productivity, which is simply output divided by labor hours. Improving labor productivity means creating more output in less time and is perhaps the central ingredient in improving living standards.

[2] By information technology, we mean electronic means of organizing and disseminating clinical or financial information.

handicap HIT installation. The large annual increases in health expenditures underline the urgency of improving healthcare productivity; otherwise, quite realistically, the healthcare system threatens U.S. economic growth. At the same time, HIT represents an enormous opportunity for improving productivity and the American standard of living.

Study Questions and Key Findings

The purpose of this study is to investigate four sets of questions.

- What is the current diffusion of HIT, especially the complex electronic health record (EHR) systems[3] that hold out the promise of healthcare transformation?
- How does EHR diffusion compare to other innovations, especially IT innovations, in other industries? And how fast will EHR likely diffuse if the healthcare system does nothing differently?
- How much would HIT diffusion likely be worth to society (1) if nothing is done differently and also (2) if adoption were quickened?
- What should the government do, if anything, to assist in the purchase or implementation of HIT and specifically EHR? Is speeding the adoption of EHR worth the costs of doing so?

Our key findings are summarized below.

- EHR is diffusing at a rate consistent with other similar IT in other industries. EHR diffusion is explicable using modern diffusion theory applicable to complex, highly networked IT products.
- Complex electronic medical records are rapidly diffusing in many segments of our healthcare system, with about 30 percent of acute-care hospital providers reporting by the end of 2003 that they had ordered EHR products and will reach 80 percent saturation in hospitals by about 2016—or earlier if assisted by the government or other organizations. Diffusion among physicians' offices is 10–16 percent, depending on the measure.

---

[3] A basic EHR system provides electronic remote user access of results in the form of text, including lab reports, radiology, transcribed notes, current medications, problems, demographics, and possibly some scanned reports. More advanced EHR systems have guideline-based content and patient- and condition-specific reminders, population management, and interprovider communication.

- The benefits of the current increase in HIT spending are arguably a *cumulative* 1 percent per year,[4] but the range varies widely depending on what else the government and healthcare players do. Other industries have shown quantifiable IT labor productivity benefits ranging from 0 percent to perhaps 4 percent per year.
- Speeding up adoption may be beneficial, although it depends on the presence of other factors such as competition and regulation. There is very strong evidence that HIT will complement these pro-productivity features. HIT is an enabler of change in how work gets accomplished. This is especially true of complex electronic medical records.
- More important than hastening adoption, which appears to have taken off since 1999 without intervention, is ensuring that appropriate incentives are in place so that complex EHRs will be used effectively.
- The U.S. federal government has the rationale, the power, and the opportunity to improve competitive conditions by promoting EHR standards, lessening network externalities at the community level,[5] and sharpening the private-market competition among providers to use the best and most efficient EHR.

Brief Overview of Research Approach

To answer the question of the current diffusion of HIT (Chapter Two), we analyzed an industry data source and compared our results to others' results. To answer the question of why HIT has diffused the way that it has (Chapter Three), we surveyed the diffusion literature to find diffusion drivers and then assessed HIT and particularly EHR on those drivers. This yielded a prediction of future EHR diffusion. To answer the question of what HIT (and especially EHR) diffusion is worth to the nation (Chapter Four), we found case studies that identified the worth of IT in other industries. We synthesized the case studies and other literature to arrive at a cross-industry theory of IT value and assessed HIT on those drivers using information from literature and interviews with providers. It is worth alerting the reader that Chapters Three and Four are not closely related analytically, but both are necessary for the analysis in Chapter Five. Finally, in asking the question of how or why should government help (Chapter Five), we started from a welfare economics perspective and attempted to identify failures in the HIT market, if any. Our review of all of the

---

[4] That is, benefits in the first year are a 1 percent increase in labor productivity, in the second year a 2 percent increase, in the third year a 3 percent increase, and so on, for as long as IT continues to change the organization of work within an industry.

[5] Network externalities will be discussed in more detail in a following chapter, but briefly: A network externality exists when a user's benefit *increases* as the number of other users increases. A fax machine is an example of an IT innovation with network externalities.

evidence from our interviews and the HIT implementation and policy literature revealed several failures, and on that basis we recommend further study of specific plausible policy interventions.

CHAPTER TWO

What Is the Current Diffusion of HIT?

We researched the current diffusion of HIT, and especially EHR, in three ways:

1. We analyzed data from Sheldon Dorenfest and Associates, a major source of HIT data. Dorenfest conducts an extensive survey of provider organizations about their IT purchases, down to the provider and vendor level. We analyzed the Dorenfest data, using our own definition of EHR that works with the data available to us. We derived a penetration curve, one provider at a time, according to our definitions.
2. We conducted a literature review of current diffusion of EHR and compared our results to those found by other authors, both in the HIT domain and in other technology diffusion domains.
3. We spoke with HIT experts and providers to gain a qualitative understanding of the HIT environment and identified barriers and enablers for HIT implementation. We used a semi-structured interview format, derived from team consensus, IT, healthcare, and management experience. Detailed results from these interviews will be reported elsewhere in 2005. The qualitative results were used as confirmatory information for the quantitative data collected in steps 1 and 2. In the discussion that follows, we report results from the interviews only when they augment what is learned in steps 1 and 2.

Results from the Dorenfest Survey

The Dorenfest Integrated Healthcare Delivery System (IHDS) database (Dorenfest database) contains information describing the overall characteristics of each integrated healthcare delivery system in the nation, as well as data about the systems' information technology programs. Dorenfest defines an IHDS as an organization that owns at least one short-term, acute-care, nonfederal hospital with at least 100 beds as defined by the American Hospital Association (AHA). This includes almost 36,000 healthcare facilities associated with 1,500 integrated healthcare delivery systems; thus a majority of U.S. hospitals are covered by this dataset. The 2003 Dorenfest database covers about 82 percent of "community" hospitals, defined in the AHA survey as "all nonfederal, short-term general, and other special hospitals." The hospitals with fewer than 100 beds not associated with a larger integrated healthcare delivery system are underrepresented in this database—about 65 percent are included compared to almost 100 percent of larger hospitals.

The data are gathered using an annual mail survey. Dorenfest asks which applications (including model and manufacturer) each IHDS has. Figure 2.1 summarizes information from the 2002[1] Dorenfest survey about adoption of clinical HIT applications. Note that adoption rates vary widely and are quite high for some applications. For example, over 90 percent of hospitals in the sample own software for labs and pharmacy.

However, our concern is diffusion of a system—an electronic health record that may provide physician order entry, guidelines, and treatment protocols and that supports patient-centered care by offering providers instant access to all clinical

Figure 2.1
Clinical HIT Software in Hospitals (2002)

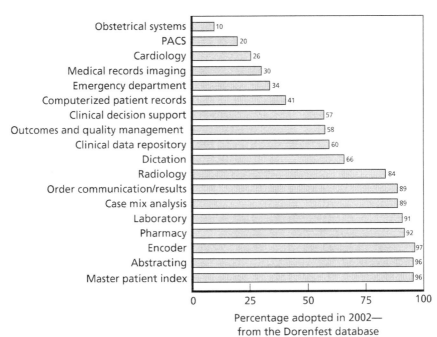

Percentage adopted in 2002—
from the Dorenfest database

NOTE: PACS refers to picture archiving and communication systems.
RAND MG272-2.1

---

[1] Please note that we use 2002 data for this figure, but that the EHR diffusion data reported below are from 2003; these data became available shortly before publication of this report.

information.[2] Dorenfest does not ask whether the facility has an electronic medical record. Therefore, we had to construct this measure from the data.

We stipulated that a provider has EHR if it has purchased *clinical decision support, computerized patient records,* and a *clinical data repository.* Authors over the years have variously defined electronic health record systems, including EHR, CPRs (computerized patient records), and the EMR-S (electronic medical record systems). Some of the terms used refer only to the patient record itself, whereas others include the entire system that supports the delivery of high-quality, integrated patient care across multiple providers. In choosing the three functions above to identify systems with an EHR, we are attempting to strike a practical midpoint in definitions as they apply to the Dorenfest data. Using these definitions, we were able to generate a diffusion curve for acute-care hospitals.

The adoption rate in physician offices is lower. Dorenfest reports that 16.4 percent of the physician offices in their dataset have EHR. Dorenfest has a large sample of over 7,800 offices, representing approximately 110,000 physicians, or roughly 22 percent of all U.S. physicians. Adoption is heavily size-dependent—adoption is 10.9 percent for sole practitioners and 37.9 percent for practices of 30 physicians or more. The overall mean is almost certainly biased upward because an office must be attached to an IHDS to be in the Dorenfest sample. Our unofficial estimate of penetration in all provider offices by the end of 2003 was roughly 12 percent.

Figure 2.2 shows the diffusion of EHR in the Dorenfest sample using our base case definition. The figure shows that, according to our definition, EHR penetration was about 32 percent by the end of 2003, which is 22 years after the introduction of the first EHR in the Dorenfest data. We also considered more conservative measures, including requiring "full implementation," not just "adopted," and requiring all three applications to be purchased from the same vendor. Requiring full implementation drops the penetration by about 6 percent, suggesting that about one in 16 offices was implementing its adopted system in 2002. Requiring two applications from the same vendor drops penetration from about 32 percent to 27 percent. The higher number seems more relevant for predicting the future, so we use the higher number.[3] This level of penetration implies, for most innovations, that it is no longer the innovators and early adopting acute-care hospitals who are adopting. The technology has reached the steep part of the uptake curve, where the "early majority" (Rogers, 1995) have begun to adopt.

---

[2] A more detailed analysis of HIT diffusion and its demographic drivers will be the subject of a future publication; only high-level results are presented here.

[3] An even better measure could be developed by mapping the reported vendor product purchase decisions into a definition of EHR. However, this would have to be done at the individual provider/product selection level and would be very labor intensive.

Figure 2.2
Diffusion of Electronic Health Records in Acute-Care Hospitals

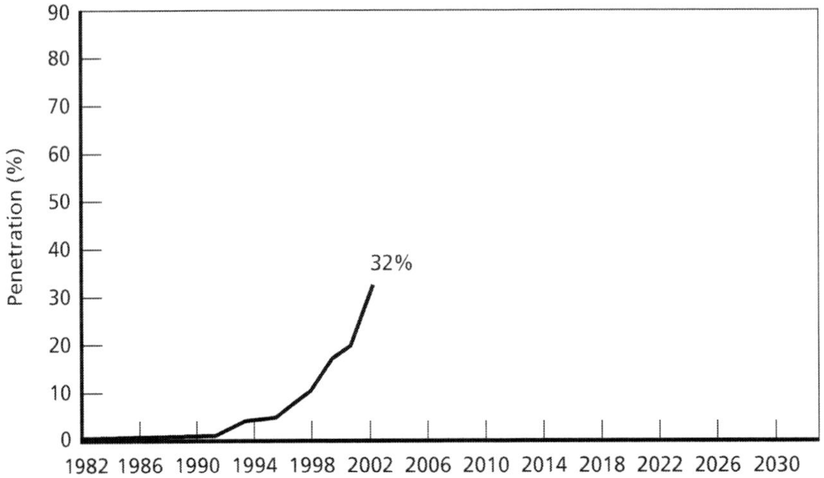

SOURCE: Dorenfest 2003 data and RAND analysis.
NOTE: n = 3,979.
RAND *MG272-2.2*

We considered potential biases of our measure. Our data record when a contract is signed, so we used that measure, even though this will overstate the true utilization rate to some extent. In addition, firms may misreport the advent of EHR if it occurred decades ago, so there is conceivably bias toward underreporting very old EHR systems. For example, the first EHR in Dorenfest by our definition occurred in 1982, although Wishard Medical Center had one by the late 1970s. Such definitional difficulties are typical with emerging technology.

We also checked our estimate of EHR penetration against others' estimates. This analysis is presented in the next section.

Review of Other Estimates of EHR Penetration

Brailer and Terasawa (2003) review the evidence on adoption of CPR and computerized physician order entry (CPOE). They note that the industry lacks a commonly accepted set of definitions and terminology for clinical information tools. There is disagreement about what functions should be considered part of CPR. We found similar problems.[4]

---

[4] EHR adoption rate measurement has some difficulties. There is a lack of clear definitions of EHR technologies and criteria for how advanced they are. Therefore, respondents' answers are often affected by an inconsistent and

With caveats duly noted, studies of adoption suggest a use rate of perhaps 22–41 percent (see Table 2.1) by the end of 2002 and perhaps 50–60 percent by 2006. However, these surveys are mostly completed by self-selected IT professionals, so the rates reported are almost certainly biased upward. Brailer and Terasawa note that five studies conducted in 2002 had an outpatient EHR use of 14–39 percent, with a median of 23 percent. However, functionality of EHR varied across the studies and the authors raise the prospect that these studies may be overgeneralizing the true rate of adoption. We found EHR adoption rates broadly consistent with the literature, although our estimate is a bit higher than others. In particular, Gartner Group suggests that only 7–10 percent of hospitals have made serious progress toward deploying CPR, and that true CPOE is closer to 1–2 percent. Data on a subset of EHRs—CPOE—had surveyed adoption rates ranging from 3.3–21 percent (Brailer and Terasawa, 2003). Yet another study, sampling at random (a preferred method), estimates complete CPOE availability at 10 percent of hospitals and partial availability at an additional 6 percent (Ash et al., 2004). As mentioned, we defined a provider as having adopted when it had signed a contract (as reported in the database), so that is likely part of the reason why our adoption rate is higher than the "deployed" EHR mentioned by Gartner. On the other hand, our estimate appears to suffer less from strong upward selection bias than others.

In summary, most of these studies have problems: The respondents are sometimes from a nonrandom sample; multiple respondents are permitted from the same organization; and one cannot always distinguish among different settings (e.g., hospital vs. ambulatory). In addition, it is rarely clear what CPR or EHR system is the focus of the study. Nevertheless, in comparing the penetration rates across studies, the

Table 2.1
EHR Adoption Levels in Other Studies

Study	Measure	Results
HIMSS (2003)	CPR system	19% fully implemented 37% in process
MIR (2001)	Computerized data record (CDR)	21.6% CDR supports some CPR 11% CDR also supports clinical codes
Modern Physician/Price Waterhouse Coopers (2003)	EMR-S	41% of respondents are from organizations that invested in EMR-S (31% in 2002)

NOTES: HIMSS (2003): n = 287 and 93 percent of respondents are Chief Information Officers; MRI (2001): n = 717 U.S. and international health professionals; *Modern Physician*/Price Waterhouse Coopers (2003): n = 436 physicians.

subjective perception of what EHR is. Also, there is no truly representative dataset of different U.S. healthcare providers giving their HIT adoption data. The Dorenfest data have these problems, although perhaps to a lesser extent than the alternatives.

RAND estimate of 32 percent for EHR adoption (from Figure 2.2) looks broadly consistent, given that we defined adoption as "contract signed." Rogers finds that adoption of innovations tends to accelerate at between 15–20 percent penetration of the population, and this seems to be certainly true with EHR as well.

Almost all of the experts we interviewed believe that there will be a sizable increase in EHR adoption in the next few years.[5] Even relatively pessimistic forecasts state that CPOE penetration will eventually top 50 percent, although not until at least 2006.

It should be noted that EHR technology is not near maturity. To take an IT example from another era, the Macintosh personal computer (PC) helped desktop computing saturate the mass market, but the computing power in that first Mac was a fraction of that in current personal computers. Certainly the future EHR will have greatly enhanced capabilities and this improvement is no doubt partly to blame for the disparate estimates of EHR penetration, as different analysts apply different technical definitions.[6]

Our examination of the available data suggests that

- EHR acute-care hospital penetration, after a 20+ year latency, might be near 32 percent by the end of 2003.
- EHR and CPOE adoption will grow significantly in the next few years. The "early majority" have begun to adopt the technology.
- The technology will improve over time. What was considered an adequate EHR today will not be considered adequate in a few years.

---

[5] In addition, some authors believe that the general perception that HIT is 10–15 years behind banking, manufacturing, and the airline industry is rapidly changing (Raghupathi and Tan, 1999).

[6] It is interesting to note that the Institute of Medicine's 2003 definition of a functional electronic health record became less ambitious in some respects than the one issued in 1991.

CHAPTER THREE

EHR Past and Future Diffusion in Relation to Other Innovations

How does EHR diffusion compare to other innovations, and how fast will it likely diffuse if the healthcare system is left alone? To answer these questions, we (1) identified historical diffusion curves, (2) surveyed the diffusion literature to identify the key drivers of diffusion, and (3) generated a prediction of future EHR diffusion based on a historical diffusion curve under a "change nothing" scenario.

Our objective was to place our project into a broader context and provide a rigorous foundation for empirically and theoretically based projections of future EHR growth. We needed a theory that would help us predict—or at least bound—EHR diffusion in hospitals and ambulatory settings if nothing were changed. We also needed to go one step further and develop a basis for predicting, or bounding, *changes* in EHR diffusion as a function of potential new government policy. This output will be used and reported on in future RAND work. In the next section, we will infer the value of this diffusion in healthcare. The review in this chapter will be structured around these goals.

Identifying Historical Diffusion Curves

We searched the literature for candidate diffusion curves and identified over two dozen. Some of the most useful for EHR can be found in Teng, Grover, and Guttler (2002), which lists the diffusion curves of 19 information technologies. The data were collected from 318 respondent firms in the United States from a mail sample of 900. The surveys asked the respondents, often chief information officers (CIOs), for implementation dates of the 19 technologies.[1] Using the survey responses, the authors constructed historical diffusion curves by adding up the number of firms that

---

[1] This method of mail survey and rely-on-recall is standard for the literature. To construct the EHR diffusion curve, we relied on self-reported adoption data from Dorenfest. The advantage of Dorenfest is that the questions are asked every year, which presumably obtains more reliable answers for recent years.

reported having adopted a technology. Some of the diffusion curves are shown in Figure 3.1. (Note that the time scales are different for the two graphs.)

Note that mainframes diffused much more slowly than PCs, and that e-mail, which began diffusing at roughly the same time as PCs, diffused much more slowly than PCs. Mainframes never diffused to 100 percent of the population, whereas Pcs eventually did so (as did e-mail, which is not shown in the figure). Computer Assisted Software Engineering (CASE) is a younger technology. Note that diffusion

Figure 3.1
Diffusion of Selected Information Technology

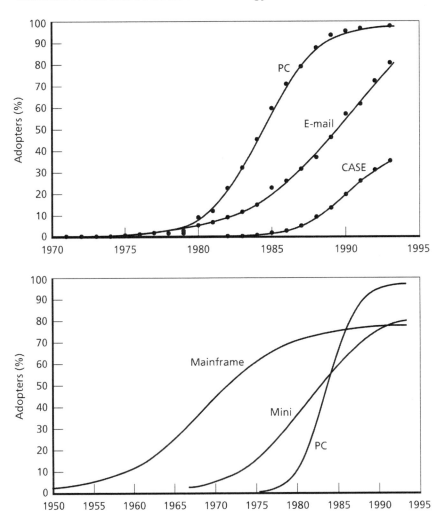

SOURCE: Teng, Grover, and Guttler (2002).
NOTE: CASE refers to computer assisted software engineering.
RAND *MG272-3.1*

speed and ultimate saturation varies within IT innovation, even for the same sample of firms.

We found consumer product diffusion curves drawn from a survey by Hall and Khan (2003). Figure 3.2 highlights the wide divergence in diffusion rates.

To compare across technologies more easily, we list the amount of time it took for an innovation to diffuse broadly across potential adopters (see Table 3.1). The table charts the time from midway through the "early adoption" period (8 percent adopted) to the end of the "late majority" period (84 percent adopted).[2]

The table illustrates that not all innovations diffuse to 100 percent of the applicable population. There are usually very good reasons for incomplete diffusion, varying from cost to technical need to technological progress of competing innovations. Also, the median adoption period, including six IT innovations, is 25 years.

Economy-wide adoption of valuable innovations—including high-value IT—can take a long time and often never reaches 100 percent.[3]

Figure 3.2
Diffusion Rates in the United States for Selected Consumer Products

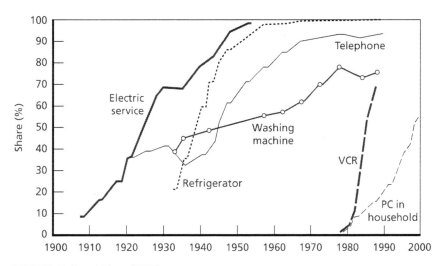

SOURCE: Hall and Khan (2003).
NOTE: VCR refers to video cassette recorder.
RAND *MG272-3.2*

---

[2] These terms are from Rogers (1995).

[3] The slowest adoption we found is the length of time it took the Royal Navy to move from clearly linking citrus consumption and the reduction in scurvy to requiring sailors to eat citrus—150 years (Rogers, 1995). There appears to be a trend over time toward more rapid adoption of innovations in general. This might suggest that more recent diffusion curves will be more relevant in understanding modern HIT diffusion. If one defines "population" broadly, then no innovation diffuses to 100 percent of the population. But more informally, it means that even those with resources and opportunity who would benefit to some extent do not always adopt the innovation.

Table 3.1
Time to Progress from "Early Adopters" to the End of "Late Majority" Is Variable

Type of Innovation	Years Taken to Diffuse to the Late Majority
Electric service	36
Telephone	> 43
Washing machine	> 60
Refrigerator	~20–30
VCR	~7
PC in households	> 15
PC in businesses	7
Mainframe	> 45
Minicomputer	~25
E-mail	11
Median	25

SOURCES: Rogers (1995); Hall and Khan (2003); and Teng, Grover, and Guttler (2002).

Drawing from the literature, we have now identified a number of candidate diffusion curves based on the history of diffusion of other innovations. EHR diffusion may resemble one of these curves, which would allow us to explain past diffusion in a general industrial context and to generate a prediction for future EHR adoption. To pick a curve, we need to have a theory to guide our choice.

Because diffusion theory is well established, we used that theory to generate a prediction of future EHR diffusion and explain its past diffusion. We provide the lessons from a large literature survey below.

Using the Literature to Identify Key Drivers of Diffusion

The diffusion literature is both vast and varied in its methodological approaches and interests. The books and articles we selected are more heavily weighted toward surveys or meta-analyses and are based on hundreds of diffusion articles and sometimes decades of research from a variety of disciplines. In our discussion, we present a condensed rather than comprehensive literature review that attempts to focus on prediction of EHR diffusion.

The literature can be organized in several categories:

Type of innovation (such as IT, agricultural, etc.).
Industry. Although healthcare is represented, a large number of industries are studied and the important theoretical results apply across industries.
Academic discipline (such as sociology, economics, etc).
Level of analysis. Level of analysis refers to whether the study attempts to understand or predict the adoption behavior of individuals, organizations, or entire industries. Individual adoption behavior, if it occurs within a firm, is often referred to as "intrafirm" diffusion.
Academic objective (such as prediction, description).

Despite the massive amount of work, most of it is descriptive, in the sense that, after collecting data on a historical diffusion process, it finds variables that are correlated with diffusion. Very little work has been performed that assists with ex-ante prediction of diffusion paths for specific technologies. This weakness in the literature appears to be increasingly well recognized, and there are now calls for further predictive work. However, there is relatively little today that is of help (with the exception of one prominent example discussed below). Partly because of this weakness, we decided to select and use important insights from several academic disciplines.[4] We found it most useful to focus on a cross-product, cross-industry, cross-disciplinary, predictive framework.

Key Papers in HIT Diffusion

The theoretically strongest diffusion papers, crucial to building a predictive theory, are outside healthcare IT. However, the key papers in healthcare IT diffusion lead us to believe that the general diffusion theory is applicable to HIT and to EHR specifically. We review below only those few papers that build the bridge from diffusion theory to healthcare IT. Where healthcare appears to specifically depart from diffusion theory, we note it in the analysis.

England, Stewart, and Walker (2000) place healthcare information technology diffusion into Rogers' (1995) well-known diffusion framework (discussed below). Their paper demonstrates that HIT can be placed in a framework that is validated by a large body of existing work. In this endeavor, the article is very much in the spirit of what we are trying to accomplish here, that is, to provide a broader context for understanding HIT diffusion. Although placing HIT into a framework is not as good as testing HIT adoption predictions in that framework, the authors are able to methodically assess variables that drive HIT diffusion. The authors conclude that the

---

[4] Furthermore, there is little work across national boundaries. Because we are concerned with U.S. HIT diffusion, we will draw more heavily from the sizeable U.S.-based literature.

observed "slow"[5] diffusion of HIT is explainable, given the providers' fragmented internal structure, immature status of strategic HIT, constrained financial resources, and complexity of the HIT systems. The authors do not attempt to predict future HIT diffusion or to suggest how government policy would change uptake quantitatively.

Anderson and Jay (1985) are important to this study because their study validates a crucial point for our purposes. They find that informal communication networks, in this case physician networks, are very important to the process of diffusion. This is consistent with Rogers' (1995) framework in which informal communication networks are important to diffusion. Anderson and Jay find that network location has a significant effect on adoption *independent* of practice characteristics or the background of a physician.

Anderson and Jay have also discovered that "epidemic effects," discussed below in more detail, play a substantial role in physician adoption: Physicians talk to each other and social interaction is an *independent* driver of adoption—it is not merely associated with the "true" variables that drive adoption.

Epidemic effects are a classic externality. Their existence in this context suggests that some government intervention to promote adoption might be socially beneficial, depending on the state of diffusion.

Having established some basic congruency between the diffusion literature and the diffusion processes inside healthcare, we turn to the broader diffusion review and methodological framework. The next two sections explain the methodology for generating a diffusion curve. Readers not interested in the technical details may skip ahead to the section titled "An Integrated Causal Model."

Generating a Predicted EHR Diffusion Curve Based on the Broader Diffusion Literature

To narrow the task of generating a predicted EHR diffusion curve, we focus on the level of analysis most important to our study: industry. This level is the most important because we are attempting to predict, or at least bound, total adoption of EHR in the healthcare *industry* over time in the United States.

However, other levels of analysis will also contribute to our understanding of diffusion, such as the Anderson and Jay (1985) paper discussed above.[6] We will also extrapolate—unavoidably—from one level of analysis to another. For example, the Anderson and Jay result pertains to individual physician behavior. We are unaware of any published analogous result for hospitals and clinics. Nevertheless, we conjecture from our site visits that some degree of epidemic effect occurs at this level, meaning

---

[5] See, for example, Dong and Saha (1998).

[6] We discuss the important issue of intrafirm diffusion at the end of this chapter. Also, the need and determinants of *effective* intrafirm diffusion permeate the discussion of the realized *value* of IT in Chapter Four.

that hospital physicians and CIOs and chief executive officers (CEOs) talk to and influence their colleagues in other institutions. Furthermore, since an industry is simply a collection of firms, we conjecture that epidemic effects operate at the industry level as well.

There are three approaches to producing a future industry diffusion curve for EHR. The first is to create a predictive, statistical diffusion model based on empirical EHR adoption data disaggregated at least to the firm level, bolstered by solid similar empirical work from other industries. The second is to generate econometrically a predicted curve based on actual EHR uptake data to date in the form of statistical extrapolation. The third is an inductive approach that picks a diffusion curve from historically "similar" industries, where a tested theoretical model guides the selection.

The first approach is preferred on methodological grounds because it would clearly link changes in policy to underlying changes in variables that drive adoption, firm by firm. Unfortunately, the first approach is infeasible. We have concluded that there is no robust predictive theory that would allow statistical estimation of EHR diffusion curves based on the multivariate model.[7] The second approach—pure extrapolation—is feasible but has been shown to be quite unreliable.[8]

We will use the third methodology. We will look for (and for EHR, have constructed from scratch) historical diffusion curves, then use diffusion theory to pick the curve or family of curves that best predict diffusion of EHR technology into the future.

To select a diffusion curve, we need to be able to describe candidate curves easily. The literature has widely used an equation to describe industry diffusion curves (see, for example, Teng, Grover, and Guttler, 2002, and Geroski, 1999). The rate of diffusion in an industry can be described as[9]

$$dN(t)/dt = (a + bN(t))[m - N(t)] \qquad (3.1)$$

---

[7] What would be required from a dataset to populate and test such a model? Just as a starting point, we would suggest longitudinal panel data of a broad sample of health providers, including their EHR adoption dates, size, for-profit status, the level of competition in each local market, products available with features and prices, government policies including subsidies and taxes, and expectations regarding future prices and features. Data on hospital marginal costs, economies of scope, and learning curves would also be helpful. Creating such a dataset is potentially feasible but has not been done yet for EHR.

[8] This method generates diffusion curves from early HIT adoption data alone. It is possible to run a regression that uses existing data to generate a "predicted" curve. It has been shown that generating diffusion curves from early adoption data is not statistically sound (Sultan, Farley, and Lehmann, 1990) because there are not enough data on which to base a reliable estimate and, perhaps more seriously, they are almost atheoretical in their construction. Thus, we will avoid relying on such estimates. Further, the adoption data are likely autocorrelated (Karshenas and Stoneman, in Stoneman 1995). While there are econometric fixes for the autocorrelation problem, they further reduce effective sample size, which exacerbates the reliability problem.

[9] A more general form of the equation that replaces the term a + bN(t) with g(t) has been used as well, but it sheds little additional light on the exposition and is omitted.

where

>   N(t) is the proportion of the total potential adopters at time t;
>   a is the coefficient of "external" influence;
>   b is the coefficient of "internal" influence or "imitation;" and
>   m is the proportion of the potential adopters that will ultimately adopt (note this may be less than 100 percent).[10]

The external influence parameter a has been interpreted as the influence of change agents such as vendors, government publicity, consultants, and so on. The internal influence parameter b could represent the influence of other adopters on the rate of adoption—notice that it is multiplied by the proportion of current adopters, $m - N(t)$. This is known in some contexts as an epidemic effect, because it is mathematically and conceptually the same as contagion models in biology, in which epidemics spread through contact among individuals. The proportion of eventual adopters is influenced by the specialization, usefulness, and speed with which an innovation overtakes it.

When this equation is fit to historical adoption curves, the statistical correlation (R^2) often will exceed 99 percent (see, for example, Teng, Grover, and Guttler, 2002, Table IV).[11] Many studies have shown that the diffusion equation (3.1) and its cousins fit diffusion data in many industries very well (Mansfield, 1961; Romeo, 1975; Sultan, Farley, and Lehmann, 1990; Wang and Kettinger, 1995). Therefore, we will use this equation in our analysis to describe diffusion curves accurately.

Typically "a" has very "low" values and "b" has much higher values. For example, the curve in Figure 3.3, drawn from the large-scale relational database technology, reflects a = 0.0006 and b = 0.31. Note the very long period between the "first adopter" at time = 0 and the technology really taking off—it takes *15 years* to progress from the first adoption to 5 percent penetration. As we discussed above, this lag is characteristic of many technologies, including IT.

The Basic Causality Problem

Because Equation (3.1) has very high levels of fit, it is tempting but completely erroneous to attribute *causality* to the model coefficients—or to go further and conclude, from the low values of "a" and high values of "b" in published regressions, that "internal" influence drives adoption. This curve characterized by Equation (3.1), or very

---

[10] Equation (3.1) is a differential equation whose solution is a logistic curve characterized by a long equation and is omitted for brevity. See Figure 3.3 for a graphical example.

[11] Other models that use a different functional form for the term a + bN(t) generate almost equally high R^2.

Figure 3.3
Diffusion Curve for Large-Scale Relational Databases

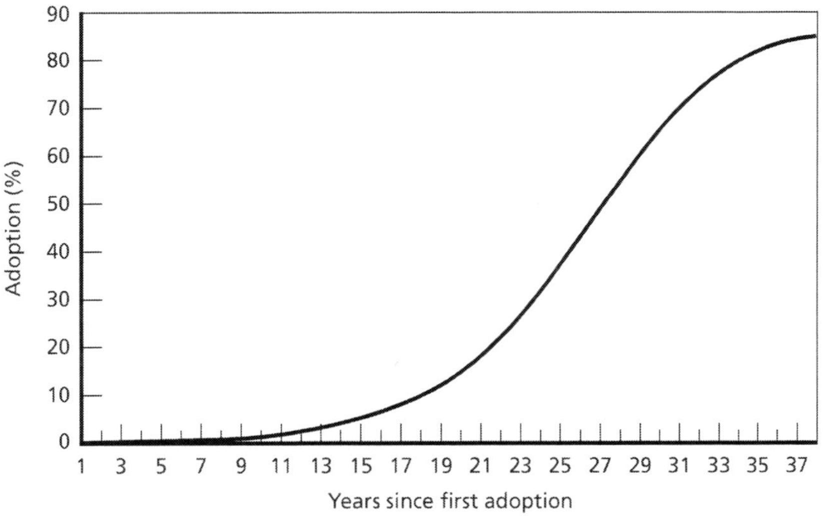

NOTE: 318 respondent firms.
RAND *MG272-3.3*

similar S-curves, can be generated by many competing theories of diffusion. For instance, a pure epidemic effect or a purely nonepidemic economic model can generate curves that fit that equation (Hall and Khan, 2003; Geroski, 1999).[12]

With more variables of microeconomic interest, a number of models have found that S-curves can be generated from adopter-level decisions in internally consistent models of individual decisionmakers (Chatterjee and Eliashberg, 1990; Chattoe and Gilbert, 1998; Silverberg, Dosi, and Orsenigo, 1988).

Because of inadequate data for micro-modeling discussed above, we will use Equation (3.1) as the basic equation for prediction but will treat it as purely descriptive—as a convenience to describe compactly and quantitatively EHR adoption behavior. Our survey of causal diffusion variables, covered next, will help us choose the correct diffusion curve.

An Integrated Causal Model

To produce our causal model, we drew from Rogers (1995), Tornatzky and Klein (1982), Moore and Benbasat (1991), Stoneman and Diederen (1994), Venkatesh et al. (2003), and O'Callaghan (in Larsen and McGuire, 1998). The resulting model therefore is our synthesis of their work, tailored to the issues of interest in this

---

[12] For example, suppose that the value of a technology is normally distributed among a population of potential adopters. Adopters never speak to each other and adopt as soon as the price drops below their valuation of the technology. Price drops linearly over time. This model will generate S-curves that will fit Equation (3.1) quite well (Hall and Khan, 2003, p. 2). Yet, by construction, there are no epidemic effects in this model.

report—for example, our interest in government policy. It is important to acknowledge the "pro-innovation" bias of most diffusion research (Rogers, 1995). We recognize that our analysis assumes that EHR will ultimately diffuse over the long run and therefore could conceivably have the same bias. However, we believe from our research that this is not a bias but, in fact, EHR's destiny. The real issue is EHR uptake speed and ultimate penetration, not whether it should or will *ever* diffuse to modern healthcare.[13]

The causal variables selected for inclusion in the diffusion model we propose are

1. Three perceived attributes of the innovation: relative advantage, compatibility, and complexity
2. External influence, such as promotion and vendor marketing
3. Social pressure via activated peer group networks (i.e., epidemic effects)
4. Network externalities
5. Degree of specialization of the innovation (i.e., narrowness of its appeal)
6. Government policy.

The sociology tradition has focused on the first three variables, whereas the economics literature has been particularly interested in the fourth. Network externalities appear to be important to adoption speed (Teng, Grover, and Guttler, 2002); Saloner and Shepard, 1995; Karshenas and Stoneman, 1993). In addition, as we discuss at the end of this report, they are very important elements of any rationale for government policy intervention.[14] The fifth variable, specialization, has not been a focus of the broad literature. However, we found that one significant paper, discussed below, predicted diffusion, and so we include it here. There is relatively less in the literature empirically on the sixth variable, government policy, although there is reasonably persuasive theory to guide us there. Some work in sociology from the 1970s details how government-led innovations can be stymied locally (Pressman and Wildavsky, 1984).

We now define each variable. We will then assess EHR on each of them and generate a predicted diffusion curve.

---

[13] However, there will be failures along the way. Southon et al. (1999) detail lessons of a failed IT initiative in a complex organization.

[14] Karshenas and Stoneman in Stoneman (1995) articulated an important alternative, economically oriented view of adoption. They view the adoption decision as an interaction between demand-side (potential adopters) and supply-side (vendor) forces. Their view is correct but not easily estimable for the same reasons already articulated: It is very data-intensive to adopt this approach and then populate the subsequent model with data. In addition, the supply side of certain HIT products, such as CPOE, is historically underdeveloped, as illustrated by the number of homegrown systems.

Definition of Causal Diffusion Variables for EHR

Perceived Attributes of the Innovation: Relative Advantage, Compatibility, and Complexity. These attributes are taken from Rogers (1995). In Tornatzky and Klein's meta-analysis of 75 diffusion studies, they found that (only) these three characteristics, among the larger set defined by Rogers, were consistently significant across those studies.

1. *Relative advantage.* Relative advantage is the degree to which an innovation is perceived as being better than the innovation that it supersedes. Relative advantage is often expressed as degree of profitability, social prestige, or other benefits.
2. *Compatibility.* Compatibility is the degree to which an innovation is perceived as consistent with the existing values, past experiences, and needs of potential adopters. An idea that is more compatible is less uncertain to the adopter and fits more closely with the organization's situation. A new idea is affected by the old idea that it supersedes.
3. *Complexity.* Complexity is the degree to which an innovation is perceived as relatively difficult to understand and use. Related to this is an innovation's "systemsness,"—more complex innovations may be adopted more slowly. A subcomponent of complexity, which is broken out separately in some studies, is trialability. Trialability is the degree to which an innovation may be experimented with on a limited basis. New ideas that can be tried piecemeal are generally adopted more rapidly than innovations that are not divisible and therefore are more complex to implement. Another complexity subcomponent is observability. Observability is the degree to which the results of an innovation are visible to others.[15]

External Influence, Such As Promotion and Vendor Marketing. Theoretically, external influences such as promotion and marketing affect adoption (purchase) behavior, although we found little evidence in the diffusion literature of promotion's effect on diffusion.[16] We found little empirical work that separates the independent effect of promotion, although almost all models mention it as a driver. In the mixed influence model, "a," the external influence parameter, is typically very small but that cannot be used to infer a low level of external influence. Because of the lack of evidence in the literature and in our site visits, we cannot use this variable when selecting a curve. Our subjective judgment is that it is not a key driver in EHR diffusion and that there are other more important factors.

---

[15] Prater and Sobol (2003) have developed a tool to estimate the profitability of IT investment in health maintenance organizations (HMOs). This is an example of a tool that increases the observability of an innovation.

[16] We did not survey the prodigious literature on the effects of promotion and advertising on purchase behavior.

Social Pressure Via Activated Peer Group Networks.[17] It is very clear from our site visits and literature review (Anderson and Jay, 1985) that physicians and hospital managers acquire adoption-relevant HIT information through informal contact with their peers. These peers are generally early adopters or "champions" of the technology and are physicians. The dissemination activities of these champions are known in the diffusion literature as "epidemic effects via activated peer group networks" (O'Callaghan, 1998).

Network Externalities. An externality is present when a cost or benefit accrues to a provider besides the purchaser. Specifically, a healthcare provider making a decision to join a network does not take into account that others will benefit from the provider's joining. For example, the Internet and the fax machine are technologies that have network externalities: purchasing an online service or a fax machine is more valuable the more other consumers can be reached with the technology. In this case, adoption may be slower than optimal, as consumers play a game of waiting for others to join first. Network externalities are prevalent in IT (Hall and Khan, 2003).

It is possible to lump network externalities under "relative advantage" above, but we treat this driver separately because of its importance in EHR for diffusion and, potentially, for government policy.

Degree of Specialization. Degree of specialization refers to the breadth of the technology's appeal. Some technologies have broad appeal for virtually all members of a population, whereas others are narrower. More specialized technologies may diffuse rapidly or slowly but will not diffuse ultimately to all potential adopters.

Government Policy. Government policy sets the rules of the game and affects incentives for adoption. We discuss government policy in detail in the policy section. Hence, we do not treat it here in our discussion of predicting EHR diffusion under the "change nothing" scenario.

Assessment of Causal Diffusion Variables with Respect to EHR

Part of our assessment relied on a series of surveys and interviews conducted at facilities that were using or contemplating the use of EHR. In the first six months, our survey used a purposive sample identified through literature and expert recommendations. The sample consisted of thought leaders and early adopters (primarily academic medical centers), new adopters of advance EHRs, primary care sites, nonadopters, and community health networks and included both closed and open healthcare systems. Sixteen sites were visited.

---

[17] Social pressure can be thought of as parts of relative advantage. We have broken them out separately because of their significance in the sociology literature and the normative theory of policy intervention discussed below.

Later visits were specifically to gather cost and HIT-related process improvement information from sites identified as engaging in these activities.

Site visits were supported by thought leader telephone interviews. The site visit goals included fact-finding and hypothesis development; identifying barriers and enablers; value measurement; and the range of implementation strategies and costs. We also met with thought leaders and early adopters to understand the state of development.

To measure firm-level attitudes, we used the key respondent approach when necessary (Hu, Chau, and Sheng, 2000), interviewing CIOs and other senior executives regarding their own organizations.[18] We bolstered the key respondent approach by interviewing other respondents in the hospital, including the CEO, nurse administrators, and other physicians. Our approach is biased toward senior officers. Therefore, our analysis may reflect adoption decisions at the organizational level more readily than the decisions of line individuals to adopt (e.g., individual physicians). We aggregated firm-level responses to obtain an industry-level assessment.[19] Finally, we relied on an extensive review of secondary sources and literature. Our summary assessment of all of this information is presented in Table 3.2.

Table 3.2
Assessment of EHR Attributes on Causal Diffusion Variables

Causal Diffusion Variable	Assessment of EHR
Perceived attributes	
Relative advantage to clinicians	High (at least, eventually)
Compatibility with existing systems of care	Moderate
Complexity (for example, is it a system or a device?)	High (definitely a system)
Other variables	
External influence	Low
Social pressure	Moderate to high—consistent with most innovations
Network effects	High
Specialization	Low to moderate
Government policy	Moderate influence to date

SOURCE: RAND site visits and secondary sources.

---

[18] The interview guide is available upon request from the author.

[19] A validated formal survey exists for individuals adopting personal workstations, which was constructed with special emphasis on generalizability to other IT adoption decisions (Moore and Benbasat, 1991). Their study is intraorganizational; our objective, in contrast, is to measure industry-level behavior.

Relative Advantage to Clinicians

Our site visits and literature review of the value of the technology indicate that although EHR is costly to learn to use, it is of high value to clinicians. This evidence will be reviewed in detail in a future report. The promise of EHR is that it will deliver high value to clinicians, if used properly. The profitability, or return on investment, of EHR has not had strong support yet. For those for whom profitability is very important, such as for-profit hospitals, adoption has been slower for EHR. This appears to reflect the lack of evidence about return on investment; this lack was revealed in our interviews of "mission"-based need to adopt EHR, and a lack of teaching hospitals in this sample. However, these adoption rate differences have been moderate in magnitude relative to other factors discussed below.[20]

We assess each variable in order below.

Compatibility with Existing Systems of Care

EHR compatibility with existing healthcare systems is moderate. We have found evidence that EHR initially impedes workflow to a minor extent, but EHR deployment does not require or cause wholesale transformation of work processes or existing power relationships in the short term. Over the long term, there may be large organizational changes. In fact, such changes are crucial to realizing the full value of EHRs, but at least initially EHR use will involve moderate changes to existing workflow or values.

The literature is consistent with this view. Eger, Godkin, and Valentine (2001) integrate IT and consumer behavior literatures to analyze the individual physician's acceptance, adoption, and application of IT. They conclude from their own review of the literature and application of their model that faster adoption will come from improved training, increased physician involvement in development, and obtaining physician buy-in before purchase. All these identified issues suggest at least some EHR resistance because of imperfect compatibility with existing systems of care.

Complexity

EHR is without question a highly complex system. This applies especially to the interoperable, complete-system vision of the future EHR. These systems take years, and millions of dollars, to implement at major hospitals, and typically tens of thousands of dollars per physician in small practices.

---

[20] In general, diffusion theory was created to explain diffusion across both profitmaking and nonprofitmaking enterprises. Health's mixed features affects but does not preclude its application here.

External Influence

As discussed above, there is little evidence to bring to bear on the variable of "external influence," such as promotion and vendor marketing, so its assessment is omitted. Our subjective judgment is that this omission is not crucial.

Social Pressure

Social pressure does not necessarily refer to coercion but generally includes peer influence. This appears to be strong in healthcare, judging by our interviews and the published literature. Physicians, especially the mainstream clinicians, often learn about new medical techniques from their peers. The early adopters tend to find information from a broader group of sources. In this sense, the diffusion of medical innovation is highly consistent with diffusion of innovations in other settings. This increases our confidence in applying a predictive model of diffusion in the next section.

Network Effects

Network effects in EHR diffusion are certainly present. Evidence rests fundamentally on the following observations: The current system is incomplete and results in duplication of tests, poorer compliance, and medical errors, among other problems. Patient care and value to the physician of any EHR are higher, often much higher, if the system has complete information at the point of care. Therefore, any provider contemplating an EHR would find the system more valuable if it can link *all* care information about its patients.

This sets up the classic externality: The value of EHR is higher if others already have it or if all providers in an area buy in at once. However, the institutional structure of U.S. healthcare is not integrated at the care level. Care is not patient-centered, it is provider-centered and operates with autonomous provider units. There may be very good, independent reasons for this decentralization, but it is hindering the integration and diffusion of EHR.

There have been notable success stories about overcoming EHR network externalities, usually involving an agency with sufficient scope to have the right incentives and an individual (almost always a physician by formal training and an IT expert by interest) who acts as an extraordinarily committed champion for digital medicine. At Inland Northwest Health Services in Washington State, this nonprofit organization created a unified EHR for more than two million patients in the region. Community physicians can access full fidelity clinical imaging, in addition to patient data, from their homes, offices, and at the point of care. Many also choose to link wirelessly. They report that the tool has decreased daily rounds by 30–45 minutes per physician.

Other authors have observed the network externality problem. Goldsmith (2003) notes that there is a physical infrastructure impediment to realizing network benefits: "because 83% of physicians' records are in paper form, building interfaces from the hospital or other physicians' offices to reach them is technically impossible" (p. 50). He also mentions mistrust between hospitals and physicians and their completely separate information domains.

Further empirical evidence, albeit indirect, for network externalities can be found in many other industries. Saloner and Shepard (1995) found fairly strong network effects in banks' adoption of automated teller machines (ATMs). Adoption is more rapid in banks with more branches (a proxy for network effects) and higher total deposits (a proxy for production scale economies). Majumdar and Venkataraman (1998) studied 40 large telecommunications firms in a dataset from 1973–1987. They found evidence for network effects but not evidence of imitative (epidemic) effects. Gowrisankaran and Stavins (2002) examined automated clearing house (ACH) technology using a quarterly panel dataset on individual bank adoption and use. They used three methods to identify network externalities. All three methods suggest that the network externalities are moderately large.

Although none of these studies in other industries proves that *EHR* has network externalities, the literature establishes that scholars have found that IT-oriented technologies in other industries have easily measurable externalities when they are looked for. The regularity of these results and others led Hall and Khan (2003) in their survey paper to single out IT as a type of innovation subject to network externalities. These findings, when combined with our healthcare-specific qualitative research, strongly suggest that there are network externalities in EHR.

Specialization

Earlier IT systems were often specialized and self contained (e.g., lab or pharmacy). However, the new EHR vision calls for integration across many clinical practices and specialties. New EHRs are meant to be used by virtually all care providers.

Selecting an HIT Diffusion Curve

In this section, we select one historical diffusion curve as a basis for predicting HIT adoption, relying on the theory and evidence presented in the previous section.

It is important to note that diffusion at the industry level (expressed as Equation (3.1)) does not connect automatically or mechanically to the data that we collect (shown in Table 3.2). To select a diffusion curve, industry-level information is needed to find parameters a, b, and m to write down the curve

$$dN(t)/dt = (a + bN(t))[m - N(t)].$$

However, what we collected is detailed qualitative site-specific information about how key informants inside their respective organizations viewed relative advantage, complexity, network externalities, and so on. Therefore, the data collected are at a different level (key respondents instead of industry) and of a different kind (characteristics instead of a, b, m). We will consider these issues in more detail in our policy analysis. Inferences will be required to make the jump from what we have to what is needed. We will use best judgment to pick a diffusion curve (a, b, m) based on specific adoption attributes listed above.

We are aware of only one paper that attempts to take characteristics from diffusion theory and use them to suggest the rate and ultimate level of diffusion (a, b, m) in an industry. We use this paper for our analysis.

As mentioned in the previous chapter, Teng, Grover, and Guttler (2002) study 19 IT applications in a survey that was sent to 900 U.S. companies and received responses from 318 firms. (This is considered a good response rate in the diffusion literature.)[21] They fit the curves to several models, finding that the model in Equation (3.1), the mixed influence model, provided the best fit in more technologies than competing models.

All the models had very high levels of fit—often over 99 percent. The 19 regressions yield 19 estimates of (a, b, m), each corresponding to one IT innovation's diffusion. Because "a" is close to zero in virtually every regression, they omit "a" and consider the pairs (b, m). They subjected the 19 pairs to a factor analysis to see how the technologies cluster. This is shown in Figure 3.4. The vertical axis is "m," the ultimate saturation, and the horizontal axis is "b," the coefficient of imitation, which is proportional to the speed of diffusion (roughly, the slope of the diffusion curve). There are similarities within the groups that appear to be explainable using diffusion theory.

According to the authors' analysis, an IT innovation will tend to achieve higher levels of saturation (high m) if it has

- High relative advantage
- Less specialized appeal/greater mass appeal
- High compatibility with user work processes
- Low complexity.

An innovation will achieve faster diffusion if

- It is a device, not a system
- Has a low level of network externalities.

---

[21] There is some evidence that mail surveys have not proven to be reliable in HIT. Ash et al. (2004) found response bias in their study of CPOE adoption.

We can now apply our assessment of EHR in Table 3.2 with the criteria immediately above. First, we consider saturation level m. EHR has high levels of relative advantage for most, but not all, practitioners. Value is relatively less to distant sites, and we hypothesize that EHR might not diffuse completely to those sites, especially if they are poorly funded. EHR has moderate compatibility, and high complexity. On balance, this implies a moderate-to-high level of ultimate saturation.

With respect to the rate of diffusion, EHR is certainly a system not a device and has significant network externalities. Taken together, this suggests a relatively slow rate of diffusion as compared to other IT innovations.

Armed with this information, we can select a candidate curve for EHR.

It appears most likely that EHR falls in Cluster 2 in Figure 3.4. That is, we might expect a large but not maximal proportion of eventual adopters and a slow rate of diffusion.

Simply inspecting the clusters in Figure 3.4, it appears that at face value EHR is a relatively good fit with Cluster 2 technologiesand a relatively poor fit with technologies in other clusters. For example, EHR requires coordination and high levels of data integration, as do large-scale relational databases (LSRDs) included in Cluster 2. On the other hand, EHR is much more complex to implement than a spreadsheet program, included in Cluster 4. (Note that spreadsheets diffused rapidly to 100 percent of the corporate population.)

We looked for a specific IT innovation to use as an EHR comparison among Cluster 2 IT innovations. These innovations included fourth generation languages (4GL), mainframes, minicomputers, and LSRDs. EHR does not appear on its face to be like a fourth generation language, so we thought that was a less likely candidate. Mainframes are over 50 years old and minicomputers are over 35 years old, and so their age may make them less of a close fit with EHR diffusion dynamics. On the other hand, LSRDs seem to be more recent and share characteristics with EHRs. Both are complex and relational and contain large amounts of data.

After this cursory review, we conducted a more in-depth comparison between EHR and a specific type of LSRD, the Enterprise Resource Planning (ERP) IT software. The two types of IT appear to share a remarkable number of similarities. See Table 3.3.

Using the above analysis, we selected the large-scale relational database curve to compare to the EHR curve. See Figure 3.5, in which the two curves are overlaid. The fit is very good. In year 22, EHR is 25 percent diffused and LSRD is estimated to be 23 percent diffused (these are regression results for LSRD, not actual numbers, but recall that the R^2 is over 99 percent). By comparison, in year 21, PCs were 99 percent diffused and e-mail was 38 percent diffused. PCs reached 25 percent diffusion—the same as EHR at end of 2002—in year 10 rather than year 21.

Figure 3.4
Cluster Analysis of 19 IT-Innovation Diffusions

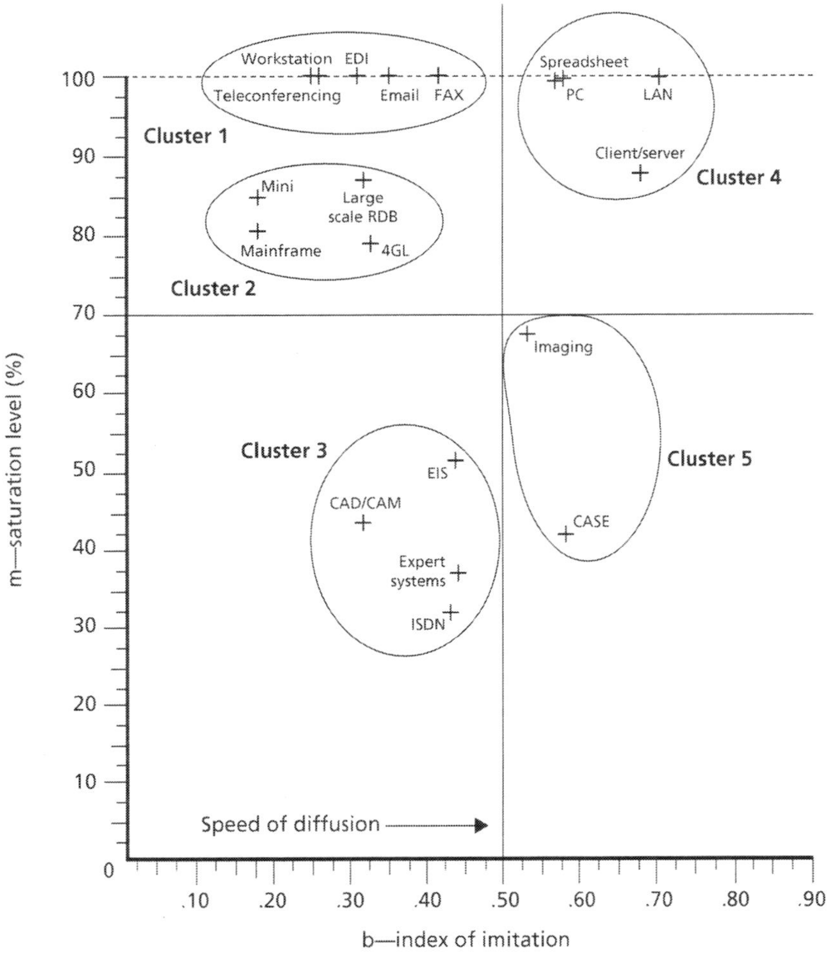

SOURCE: Teng, Grover, and Guttler (2002).
RAND *MG272-3.4*

The definitional difficulties of assigning the date for the first EHR (discussed in Chapter Two) could move the EHR curve in Figure 3.5 to the left by a few years, which would change the point estimates for the curve and make it look like a less perfect fit. Also, physician office diffusion is lower, as noted above. However, note that the general shapes of the curves are very similar. For purposes of future prediction, given current penetration, the starting date is less important than the overall shape and ultimate saturation of the diffusion curve.

Table 3.3
Comparison of Enterprise Resource Planning and Electronic Medical Record IT

Point of comparison	ERP	EHR
Objective	Integrate and optimize an enter-prise's internal manufacturing, finan-cial, distribution, and human resource functions	Integrate and optimize a care provider's physicians, financial operations, labs, and pharmacy
First steps in implementation	Complex and expensive re-engineering of legacy IT systems	Complex and expensive re-engineering of legacy IT systems
First generation technology	Intrafirm collaboration among de-partments	Intrahospital collaboration among departments
Second generation tech-nology	Collaboration across firms (e.g., ven-dors)	Collaboration across care provid-ers (e.g., hospitals and physicians' offices)
Information flow	Real time and simultaneous	Real time and simultaneous
Consequences of inaction	Department or firm isolated within its business environment	Department or care provider iso-lated within its care environment
Based on the above . . .		
Complexity	High	High
Network externalities	High	High

SOURCE: Gartner Group and RAND analysis.

Figure 3.5
Diffusion of EHR LSRD

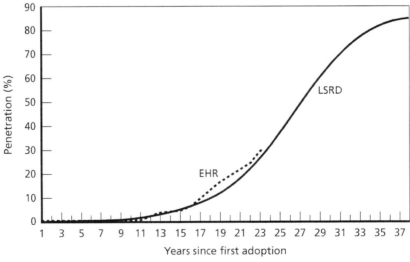

In light of these results, it seems that EHR diffusion has been "slow" more with respect to high expectations of innovators than with respect to historical rates of diffusion across numerous technologies, including recent IT innovations. In addition, to the extent that it has been slow, it is explainable within classic diffusion theory—historically, complex systems diffuse more slowly and systems characterized by externalities diffuse more slowly. EHR has both of these qualities.

Considering both theory and historical information, it may not be realistic to expect EHR to diffuse across 100 percent of potential adopters without government intervention.

The literature has less to say about why diffusion in an industry starts at a specific time. Because of the long latency, another question might be why does IT diffusion in healthcare rapidly increase later than in other industries? Without much theory available, we will allow ourselves some speculations. First, diffusion by type of HIT varies dramatically—in contrast to EHR, financial or stand-alone applications have diffused widely and early in healthcare. These applications had a direct effect on institutions' financial health, and adopters took advantage of them. Second, comparisons to other industries tend to suffer from selection bias; healthcare is compared to those industries in the vanguard of IT implementation. It might be more fair to compare it to the median industry. Third, as England, Stewart, and Walker (2000) pointed out, EHR is slower because it is a complex, networked product that is being introduced into a very complicated and uncoordinated system. The barriers that this lack of coordination causes will be discussed in more detail in the next two chapters.

Note that we might expect 80 percent diffusion of EHR by year 33, or roughly 2016, even without intervention by the government. We thus should expect EHR to diffuse broadly, although not maximally, to the provider population. We now turn to the question of how much broad EHR, and HIT, diffusion might be worth to the U.S. economy.

CHAPTER FOUR

The Potential Value of Wide HIT Diffusion

How much might HIT be worth in the long run? What magnitude of productivity gains is available? If HIT diffuses broadly, in particular if EHR diffuses broadly and transforms healthcare, what might society expect to gain? To answer these questions, we must first return to the broader term of HIT, rather than considering EHR alone, even though EHR is almost certainly the most important part of the investment and one that will be largely completed over the next 15 years.

We use two complementary methodologies to answer the question of HIT value—"bottom-up" and "top-down." The bottom-up method is a deductive, micro-level approach based on results from generally peer-reviewed medical journals. It has the advantage of clearly linking gains from studies of specific HIT interventions for particular populations to overall gains, and allows HIT gains to be identified by stakeholder. This approach will be discussed in forthcoming research. We employ the complementary, top-down approach for reasons discussed below.

There are problems with using the bottom-up approach to measure the longest of the long-term gains. HIT is a complementary product that helps enable long-term work flow changes. Journal articles report (generally speaking) short-term results because the HIT innovations studied are new in the reporting organizations. Furthermore, even if the HIT innovation is not new, it is very difficult to attribute long-term changes to any one innovation. Therefore, the bottom-up approach cannot easily forecast the truly large gains that the work flow changes might enable. These changes may take a decade or more to show up. What is needed is evidence regarding long-term changes and productivity gains and a theory of the drivers of IT benefits.

Such evidence exists in other industries. Some industries have undergone this IT transformation and obtained major productivity benefits, resulting in higher profits, higher wages, and, especially, higher consumer surplus. Other industries have made the IT investment but have not reaped the benefits.

We study both types of industries to understand inductively the magnitude of the gains and the complementary activities or factors that must take place to realize long-term gains from HIT. We then assess healthcare on those activities and factors, using literature reviews and site interviews. This generates a range of predictions for the value of HIT.

It is worth noting that this chapter is not closely related analytically to Chapter Three. The specific diffusion curve identified in Chapter Three does not alter the analysis here. In Chapter Three, we picked a specific diffusion curve for EHR; in this chapter, we explore what rapid IT diffusion has been worth in other industries. However, both chapters are necessary to inform the policy discussion and conclusions in Chapter Five.

But first, since we will need to discuss productivity to discuss value, we turn our attention to the issue of measuring productivity in healthcare.

Measuring HIT Productivity Improvements in Healthcare

HIT productivity benefits will likely arrive in the form of higher quality and lower costs. At its simplest, productivity is output divided by input. For example, quality adjusted life years (QALYs) divided by labor hours could be a candidate measure of healthcare labor productivity. Many successful healthcare innovations are aimed at making people healthier, at some (hopefully small) incremental cost. How would such an innovation affect labor productivity? In this case, the input (cost, in the denominator) goes up, but the numerator (QALYs in this example, in the numerator) goes up more. Overall, productivity (the ratio) goes up.

One problem with health productivity statistics has been the difficulty of measuring output at the national, aggregated level. Historically, there have been some poor measures of productivity. In some instances, inputs to production were used as proxies for outputs.[1] This ensures a measured productivity gain of zero.

Ultimately, if HIT is valuable, it should be cost effective and deliver more QALYs per dollar of healthcare spending. For example, if HIT reduces medication errors without additional labor, that will reduce morbidity and mortality (increasing QALYs) and lower costs by avoiding additional expenditures to treat the iatrogenic illness. This would increase productivity.[2] There are also process measures of quality, and HIT, with its emphasis on clinical decision support and best practice guidelines, will certainly help improve performance on those measures.

In the following analysis, some care was taken to choose industries in which the productivity statistic is reasonably well measured. Difficulties still remain, which will be dealt with in the case analysis. For example, productivity increases sometimes

---

[1] For example, bed days was used at one point to measure healthcare output.

[2] If healthcare were a standard or textbook industry, economics would assert that the productivity benefits of added health and higher quality could be collected by charging higher prices that reflect what people are willing to pay for better health. It is a market failure that healthcare providers can do so only very imperfectly. We will discuss this in more detail in Chapter Five.

years after the initial investment. Productivity in the short run may decrease. Also, firms may increase efficiency without increasing investment, which will show up as increased productivity.

There is another measurement difficulty besides measuring productivity. It is difficult to attribute productivity gains to HIT specifically, as opposed to complementary changes in healthcare inputs, such as labor mix, physical plant, and mediating variables (e.g., work processes). This same difficulty will be seen in studies in other industries. However, that does not make the analysis useless at all; on the contrary, it points us in the direction of understanding the broader process changes and complementary investments that must take place *in addition to HIT investment* to obtain large gains. In summary, while productivity is the right type of measure, the specific productivity measure must be chosen and interpreted with care.

One additional investment that must take place is effort in implementation. The time that it takes to perform excellent implementation is part of the reason why IT benefits usually take time to appear. We briefly review this literature before turning to the studies of HIT value.

Implementation—A Key Factor in Realizing HIT Value

So far, we have not discussed the important issue of effective and widespread diffusion within the firm and the implementation techniques that assist this process. However, we have found that it is a very important issue for HIT. It is important because it has been shown that the ultimate value of HIT depends on much more than whether an organization adopts it. It depends directly on how many doctors in a practice use it and how often they use it and how well (Miller and Sim, 2004). Ultimately, potential users must use HIT to get the value out of it. With respect to EHR, because it is networked, the value (meaning lower costs, better quality, and fewer deaths) increases faster than the number of users. Because of the importance of getting all potential users to employ EHR, lessons from the implementation literature are particularly relevant.

The implementation literature has found that three factors are key to successful implementation: (1) the properties of the innovation (such as compatibility and complexity); (2) the features of the organizational context (such as size, degree of centralization, political and regulatory constraints, and orientation toward change); and (3) the characteristics of the implementation strategy (that is, the series of activities realized in the day-to-day work practices of the targeted context, Bikson et al., 1995). In a study of the early 1980s implementation of office technology, Bikson found that "resistance to computer use" was *not* a key factor in implementation (Bikson, 1987). This finding is reaffirmed 20 years later in our literature reviews and other research into physician EHR use.

In our site visits, we saw that all three of these factors matter a great deal with respect to EHR implementation success. In particular, the third factor, implementation strategy, including buy-in of medical staff and adequate IT support and training, is crucial to success. Also, the features of the organizational context have predicted success—very decentralized providers have tended to have more trouble with EHR implementation.

Other studies reinforce the finding that gains from the innovation increase in the commitment to implementation. In another study of an IT innovation, payoffs to implementation of Electronic Data Interchange (EDI) varied in proportion to its embeddedness within the organization (Chatfield and Yetton, 2000). In this case, embeddedness is defined as the degree to which an EDI network is central (rather than peripheral) to managing interfirm interdependence.

EHR is intended to be absolutely central to managing such interdependencies. It should be *the* coordinating device for patient-centered care. Thus, the implementation literature suggests that marginalizing EHR, allowing workarounds, or creating off-line communication mechanisms among providers will severely reduce its value. Our site visits and visits with experts certainly confirm this insight.

Other important success factors, identified by Bikson et al. (1997) and echoed in our site visits to providers with EHR, are planning for implementation, addressing a genuine user need, using pilot projects, eliciting strong support from senior management (including medical management), and choosing vendors with practical experience.

In a landmark study of software implementation, The Standish Group (1995) found that a shocking 31 percent of software projects (with a median expenditure of $2.3 million for a large company) failed. After extensive case studies, they identified the following variables as critical to the success of implementation:

- User involvement
- Executive management support[3]
- A clear statement of requirements
- Proper planning
- Realistic expectations.

There is adequate evidence that the same criteria apply to successful implementation of EHR.

Our discussion of the value of EHR implementation below assumes that successful implementation techniques are applied with some diligence within providers. Implementation skills are crucial to realizing the value from the HIT investment.

---

[3] Also, see Goldsmith (2003), p. 173.

The reader may ask, why make the assumption that implementation is handled well? Although implementation is very important and often is not handled well, the next chapter concerns itself with the potential value of HIT. If implementation is poorly handled, we already know that the value of an HIT investment will be close to zero, or negative. By ignoring implementation analytically, we can establish an informal upper bound on the value of HIT. Furthermore, in the long run, competition should force effective implementation of valuable innovations. Since this analysis forecasts the long run, assuming efficient implementation in the long run may be the most appropriate perspective. There is also some empirical support for this assumption: Many initial ERP implementation failures are followed by a second and more successful trial.[4]

We now return to the top-down analysis of HIT's potential long-term value. There are two types of IT productivity evidence: macroeconomic and microeconomic. Macroeconomic evidence considers evidence of IT benefit in the entire U.S. economy taken as a whole. Microeconomic evidence considers IT benefit realized in specific industries. We consider the macroeconomic literature and then the (more persuasive) microeconomic literature.

Benefits of IT in the Overall U.S. Economy and in Specific Industries

Benefits of IT in the Overall Economy

Massive IT investment took place in the U.S. business community in the 1980s. A PC was put on almost every work desk, as reflected in the PC diffusion data in Figure 3.1. Supply chain management was automated, and customer data in a large number of industries were computerized.

By the mid-1990s, annual U.S. labor productivity increases continued to lag noticeably behind many other national economies. Investigations were launched, and one main culprit was identified: information technology. People started to ask: Where are the economic gains for our billions of dollars of IT investment? There was talk of overinvestment, or at least underuse, of IT.

By the late 1990s, the story had changed. U.S. productivity surged in the second half of the 1990s. After some investigation, many concluded that IT investment was finally showing up in national productivity gains.[5] Oliner and Sichel (2000) find that IT created an extra 0.7 percent per year increase in labor productivity (see Figure 4.1). The gains accumulate over time. Furthermore, most of the evidence from recent

---

[4] Personal communication with J. Teng, University of Texas, September 2004.

[5] See for example, Jorgenson and Stiroh (1999).

Figure 4.1
IT Is Now the Single Biggest Driver of Increases in U.S. Labor Productivity

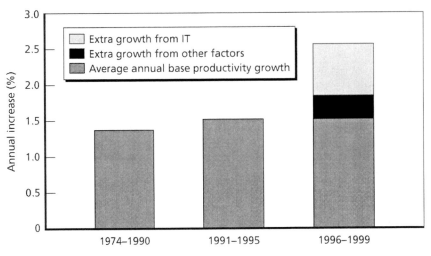

SOURCE: Oliner and Sichel (2000).
RAND *MG272-4.1*

government statistics suggests that the gains of the late 1990s have continued into the early 2000s.

The result that IT contributes such a large proportion to growth is not without controversy among growth accounting economists. It is well known that in economic booms, as occurred in the late 1990s, output increases faster than labor hours; therefore labor productivity improves. Exactly how much of the increased labor productivity to attribute to this cyclicality varies by study. If one attributes a great deal of a productivity increase to cyclicality, that leaves less for IT to explain.

One notable exception to the bullish consensus is Gordon (2002), who analyzes aggregate growth data and finds that almost all of the growth is due to cyclical factors. However, most studies find some solid improvements to labor productivity in the late 1990s, with a sizable fraction due to IT. More recent Bureau of Labor Statistics data, through 2003, seem to strongly confirm this: Productivity has continued to improve markedly even without strong economic growth. It appears to be a major factor in the "jobless recovery" of 2002–2003.

The suggested reasons for the delay in realized productivity improvements were that firms have to learn how to use IT to re-engineer their work processes and have to get enough IT on board to realize the benefits of IT complementarities. There appeared to be perhaps a 5–15 year lag between the IT investment and large labor productivity gains. In other words, there is a long latency between investment and return.

However, relying on nationally aggregated growth data is not adequate for our purposes, partly because it includes productivity numbers from IT industries *them-*

selves, which are not relevant. The productivity improvements of *using* IT in a non-IT-producing industry (e.g., health) are conceptually different from the productivity improvements *within* an IT-producing sector (e.g., computers or microprocessors). We would want to ignore gains in IT-producing sectors.

In addition, Bureau of Labor Statistics data clearly show that the productivity gains were not uniform across industries, so how one slices the data matters. This variation raises the obvious question of whether healthcare would be one of the star users of IT or one of the laggards—many non-IT-producing industries had no productivity gains at all.

A McKinsey Global Institute (MGI) study (2001) establishes the barely positive and statistically insignificant overall relationship between IT investment growth per employee (called the capital intensity growth rate) and acceleration in productivity growth, no doubt partly a result of latency effects.

The reason for this can be seen by charting the industries according to how much they contributed to the late 1990s growth acceleration. In fact, only six industries (31 percent of GDP) constituted 99 percent of the productivity growth increase of 1.33 percent from the early to the late 1990s. Figure 4.2 depicts net growth and identifies the largest contributing industries, many of which will be discussed below. The figure shows that very large productivity gains have recently been rather concentrated in a few industries. Whereas a solid 65+ percent of the economy grew at least a

Figure 4.2
Cumulative Productivity Contribution Diagram: 1995 Productivity Growth Jump

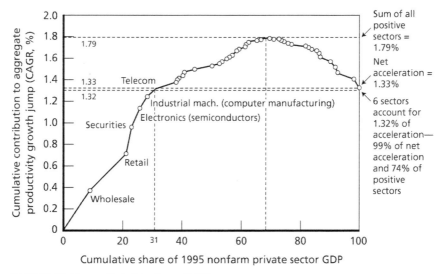

SOURCE: McKinsey Global Institute (2001).
NOTE: CAGR refers to compounded annual growth rate.
RAND *MG272-4.2*

little, roughly 35 percent of the economy suffered lower productivity. Besides raising questions about measurement error, this suggests that specific industry factors drive growth.

In summary, macroeconomic growth data show a weak correlation between IT intensity and productivity growth in general, at least in the short term. In addition, an analysis such as ours requires that we exclude IT-producing industries. Macroeconomic growth data also lack any explanation of industry-level factors, including government policies, that may have contributed to productivity results. Therefore, we need to look at microeconomic data from other industries to understand potential HIT benefits for healthcare.

Benefits of IT in Specific Industries

The only healthcare productivity analysis that we uncovered was an MGI study comparing healthcare productivity across several countries; the study did not focus on IT. The productivity literature in health is sparse, no doubt partly because of the difficulties in measuring healthcare productivity. Therefore, we review analyses of other industries and draw lessons from those for healthcare.

Stiroh (2002) poses the question: "IT and the US productivity revival: What do the industry data say?" He finds that productivity gains from IT are broad-based—averaging a solid contribution of 0.92 percent per year in the noncomputer sectors in the economy. However, McKinsey reports that if Stiroh had removed all six of the highest-performing sectors, rather than only the four that he did remove, then the gains would have evaporated. In other words, it is possible that the productivity gains are not broad-based in the noncomputer sectors.

Figure 4.3 depicts the number of sectors of the economy that experienced a productivity growth jump of at least 3 percent in the six years surrounding 1995. (Three percent was an arbitrary but seemingly reasonable number chosen by MGI as a cutoff for being economically significant.) The number is pro-cyclical and varies between two and 11. The most recent period, which includes the productivity renaissance in question, had a very average eight sectors with that improvement. The number of sectors with productivity growth jumps was not unusual and therefore not especially broad-based. Instead, the unusual feature of the late 1990s is the large size of the high-performing sectors, reflected in the share of employment in the "jumping" sectors. In particular, the enormous retail and wholesale sectors were two sectors that enjoyed great productivity growth. The size of the sectors helps partly to explain why aggregate U.S. productivity did so well in the period.

Figure 4.3
Number of Sectors with Growth Acceleration of at Least 3 Percent

Number of jumping sectors[a]

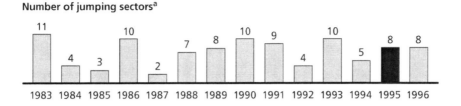

1983 1984 1985 1986 1987 1988 1989 1990 1991 1992 1993 1994 1995 1996

% share of employment in jumping sectors[a]

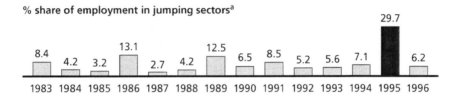

1983 1984 1985 1986 1987 1988 1989 1990 1991 1992 1993 1994 1995 1996

SOURCE: McKinsey Global Institute (2001).
[a]A sector is classified as "jumping" in year Y if its compounded annual growth rate of productivity for years Y through Y+3 is at least 3 percent higher than it was for years Y–3 to Y.
RAND MG272-4.3

MGI conducted an extensive study of the drivers of productivity gains, with special emphasis on understanding the source of productivity growth in IT-intensive industries. The industry data showed that some IT-intensive industries had not grown faster than average, whereas others had. MGI chose a number of high-IT-investment industries to examine in case studies to identify the sources of growth. They chose to study both high-performing and low-performing industries and IT-producing and IT-using industries.

From this sample, RAND chose to review the non-IT-producing cases, because these would be the most similar to healthcare, given that it does not produce IT. We considered six cases: telecommunications, securities trading, retail (including general merchandising), wholesale, retail banking, and hotels.

Three Categories of IT Investor Industries
We judged how successful these firms were in capitalizing on their IT investment and assigned them to one of three categories:

1. Dramatic successes (telecommunications, securities trading)
2. Successful users (retail, wholesale)
3. Disappointments (hotels, retail banking). (See Table 4.1.)

Table 4.1
IT Productivity Gains Varied by Industry

Industry	Annual Productivity Gains, 1995–1999	Output Measure (Input Measure Is Always Labor Hours)	Amount Roughly Attributed to IT
Dramatic Successes			
Telecommunications	8%	Local access lines and call minutes + mobile subscriptions and mobile minutes + long-distance calls	Substantial—but only a complement to other factors
Securities	18.9% in nonportfolio management	# equity trades plus deflated $ value of underwriting deals	Substantial—but only a complement to other factors
Successful Users			
Wholesale	8.2%	Value added	1–3%
Retail	6.3%	Value added	1–2%
Disappointments			
Retail banking	4.1%	No. of various transactions	0% to negative
Hotels	0%	Quality-equivalent room nights sold	0%

As a way to make comparisons to the national economy, keep in mind that the overall gains for the economy from 1995–1999 from IT have been estimated at 0.7 percent per year and for the noncomputer sector were 0.9 percent per year (with a wide variance by industry).

All these industries had high growth rates in IT investment in the late 1990s, generally in the 12–18 percent range per year per employee. (This will be discussed in more detail below.)[6] But they had very different productivity outcomes. Our discussion below is intended to help develop insight about what we might expect HIT to deliver in healthcare and what the key drivers of success are. These insights will also help to inform the policy discussion in the next chapter.

Telecommunications. A series of interrelated events propelled the telecommunications industry to 8 percent annual productivity growth over a period of 12 years (and likely continuing into 2005). The events occurred in a specific beneficial order. Deregulation stimulated massive competition in the industry. On the technical engineering side, the carrying capacity of a single fiber increased 230 percent *per year* for

---

[6] One other reasonable figure to use might be, for example, marginal investment per employee. However, the MGI analysis used the growth rate, so marginal investment is not readily available. Also, growth rates rather than dollar figures also provide a common reference for industries that vary enormously in IT capital per employee.

six years in a row. This in turn led to high investment in capacity to deliver phone minutes, especially mobile phones. The capacity plus the competition stimulated large price decreases by carriers for consumers. The large price decreases greatly increased demand for phones and minutes. Finally, the telecommunications industry was able to respond to the demand for more minutes without adding workers in proportion to the minutes. This led to the 8 percent annual increase in labor productivity. (Note that increased demand led to the productivity improvement. Thus, operating at an efficient scale, at high-capacity use, is an important productivity driver.)

MGI does not attempt to isolate the *independent* effect of IT in productivity growth; indeed, it is probably not possible to do so. IT clearly enabled growth. Without the IT capacity backbone, growth would have been much lower. But without competition to stimulate investment in capacity and price decreases, productivity growth would have been much lower. In addition, deregulation helped to enable the competition to take full advantage of the technical progress.

In the telecommunications industry, one can think of competition, deregulation, and IT as economically complementary factors—the whole is truly greater than the sum of the parts. When this is true, the gains of any one complementary ingredient are not determined, in the same way that a bolt's value is dependent on the presence of a nut. In telecommunications, it is the sum of all three factors (competition, deregulation, and IT) that created the spectacular productivity outcome.

In this case, a fixed IT capital infrastructure was put in place that could handle increased demand without adding workers.

Securities Trading. Securities trading is one of the very few industries in the late 1990s where the Internet had an effect on industry productivity. The Internet helped to create online trading, which led to brokerage staff reductions. There was also increased competition, partly because of deregulation and partly because of continued pressure from discount brokerages such as Schwab. As with telecommunications, IT installed an infrastructure that allowed more trades at minimal cost.[7] When securities trading skyrocketed during the late 1990s stock market bubble, labor did not increase very much.

The result was that labor productivity went up by a remarkable 18.9 percent per year. Some of the gains were given back in the early 2000s, when trading dropped after the Internet bubble burst.

MGI concluded that the productivity increase came from the combination of growing demand, deregulation, competition, and IT. Clearly, the booming stock market rapidly drove up the volume of trades and the dollar value of deals and this had a major effect on productivity. Of course, it is cyclical. However, gains in the

---

[7] Presumably, this will decrease the value of an individual trade, all things equal. This lowers the value per trade. Overall, value should go up. This may be similar to what will happen with e-visits in health: more value, but less value per e-visit than with a classic doctor visit.

early 1990s were still strong, so it is not entirely cyclical. Because of the cyclicality and churning, securities is a bit harder to apply directly to healthcare.

In summary, the dramatic productivity successes in IT in the U.S. economy were telecommunications and securities trading. Note that these dramatic successes are in technology-heavy businesses that found a way to increase demand and strongly leverage technology. For example, it was possible to use IT to allow mobile phone minutes to grow without increasing labor proportionally.

IT can enable an industry to build infrastructure that allows future increases in demand or increases in quality (value added) to take place without further increases in labor. IT may not substitute for labor in the short run but is often an enabler of future growth at much lower marginal cost than before.

Below we will look at whether such conditions could exist in healthcare in the first part of the 21st century. The "successful users," whom we survey next, require more bricks and mortar and more personal contact to make sales. In this regard they appear to be more like healthcare.

Retail, Including General Merchandising Services (GMS). Retail includes GMS, which includes Wal-Mart, Target, and other big box stores. The retail sector saw productivity growth of 6.3 percent in 1995–1999, whereas IT investment grew at an 18.9 percent rate per employee annually.

This growth rate is attributed to several factors. There was increased competition in the segment, with a strong champion for change (Wal-Mart) that placed pressure on itself as well as on its competitors. Almost literally, there was a "Wal-Mart effect" in general merchandising, with the chain driving itself and its competitors to higher and higher levels of efficiency.

An additional contributor to the boost in productivity in the late 1990s was the move of consumers to higher value-added goods. This is partly a cyclical phenomenon, as confident consumers in the late 1990s substituted more expensive for less expensive goods. This shows up in the productivity statistics as increased value added for the same amount of labor. This phenomenon does not appear to be IT-related.

There were significant IT-enabled changes, including more extensive use of cross-docking[8] enabled by electronic supply chain tools; use of forecasting tools to better align staffing levels; and improvements in use rates at checkout.

MGI estimates that about 15–35 percent of the increase was due to IT. The willingness to place some bound on the independent value of IT in retail stems from the fact that, in contrast to the dramatic successes, fewer of the improvements appeared to be entirely complementary. Also, the different sector reports probably had different authors.

---

[8] Cross-docking means to take a finished good from the manufacturing plant and deliver it directly to the customer with little or no handling in between.

For lack of a better statistic, we will use this 15–35 percent contribution estimate for wholesale as well.

Retail and general merchandising had strong growth, partly because of increased competition and a productivity champion in Wal-Mart, but the sector took advantage of available IT solutions to improve business processes. It was not a panacea, but IT had an effect and enabled change in a highly competitive sector.

Wholesale. This vast and complex sector of the economy posted huge 8.2 percent annual productivity gains from 1995–1999, and a 5.3 percent productivity jump compared to 1987–1995. Wholesale increased IT per employee by a solid 16.9 percent per year in the period, up from 12.7 percent in 1987–1995. Wholesale, like retail, used IT to boost efficiency. Foremost among the IT innovations was increased warehouse automation. Also, a great deal of industry consolidation helped to spread best practices, including best IT practices.

However, other labor-saving innovations were not IT-related. Those included the move toward higher value-added products (induced by the retailers) and improved stock-picking techniques. However, one could conclude that the judicious use of IT helped make business processes run better. The type of IT gains were somewhat similar to those within retail, so applying the same percentage contribution of IT, one arrives at a contribution of IT of 1–3 percent per year.

In summary, heavy competitive pressure, combined with IT, led the "successful users" to impressive 6–8 percent annual productivity improvements per year, and about 2 percent annually can be attributed to IT directly. We will assess the usefulness of these results in the healthcare context below.

We now turn to the IT "disappointments."

Hotels. Hotels made a large IT investment in the late 1990s, as did the dramatic successes and the successful users. IT investment grew at an 11 percent annual rate from 1995–1999, five times faster than that in the 1987–1995 period. Specifically, there was a substantial investment in customer relationship management software and pricing software. The intent was to improve and expand on existing customer relationships and target customers for customized marketing.

However, the IT investment was underused. Hotels were making very large profits during the economic boom, especially in large urban markets, since the supply of hotel rooms is fixed in the short run. Hotels did not feel pressure to use the IT investment to its utmost. (The excess revenue from price increases caused by room shortages needed to be accounted for and backed out of the analysis, similar to the retail and wholesale sectors.)

It is interesting to note that in the past the hotel industry had a better track record in using IT. For example, the highly valuable investment in booking software was made in the late 1980s, which allowed booking agents in remote locations to have instant access to accurate vacancy information. This prevented agents from telling prospective customers that rooms were sold out, when in fact there were rooms available in other niches of the system. These IT gains had already been realized by 1995.

Therefore there is evidence that IT-led productivity gains not only vary by industry, but also by time period and specific IT application.

It is notable that over 50 percent of hotel staff are maids and janitors, who are relatively unaffected by IT. Overall, the effect of IT on productivity growth in hotels in the late 1990s was judged to be negligible. It is interesting to note that healthcare, especially hospitals, have substantial hotel-like functions and could likely have some of the same problems in leveraging IT for a segment of their employees.

Retail Banking. Retail banking, like hotels, was an IT productivity disappointment. Productivity grew at a reasonable rate of 4.1 percent during 1995–1999, but this was 1.4 percent slower per year than in the previous eight years. From 1995–1999, banking made a large IT investment, growing IT investment by 16.8 percent per employee per year, up from 11.4 percent in 1987–1995. For example, banking invested in an average of two computers per employee in the four-year span.

However, interviews revealed that these computers did not deliver big productivity gains because the average employee did not really need the functionality and computing power in the new machines. The expensive functionality sat on the desktops without transforming the business. Banking, like hotels, invested in customer relationship management software, but it was judged mostly a failure. The data were not used nor marketing strategies devised to exploit the new information (although it is noted that they may be exploited in the future). It was also felt that mergers disrupted investment and that IT-enabled product proliferation did little to improve customer relations or bank profitability. Finally, the successful implementation and use of ATMs had largely occurred before 1995 and so did not contribute to further productivity improvements after 1995.

The customer relationship management "failure" reported above points out an apparent weakness in the MGI methodology that is not easily remedied. As we noted in the discussion above, IT gains can have a latency of over 10 years. Therefore, growing current IT investment (one of the selection criteria of MGI) may not lead to high productivity until years later, thus leading to a spurious negative correlation between high current growth in IT spending and current productivity growth. So it appears that the MGI methodology is not completely consistent with results from other literatures that suggest long latency. We note that this is a weakness, but it is mitigated by the ability of detailed case studies to draw firmer conclusions about work process changes and cause-and-effect relationships in general.

Not all banking IT in this period was a failure. Imaging and voice recognition delivered gains, as imaging contributed to faster transmission and recording of checks, and customer relations staff were replaced by voice recognition.

Online banking was an innovation in the 1990s. Online banking could decrease staff time per transaction, but online banking penetration in 1999 was so low that it did not affect aggregate banking labor productivity. There is also a productivity measurement problem: the customer convenience in online banking is an unmeasured benefit, at least when productivity is measured as the number of transactions.

Finally, like hotels, banking was profitable in the late 1990s, largely because noninterest income from stocks and property buoyed profits. This eased competitive pressures.

In summary, there was a slackening of labor productivity improvements, and underused IT contributed to this slackening.

Information Technology as a Competitive Weapon

In all of the cases where IT contributed to high productivity, it was seen and used as a *competitive weapon* for differentiating a firm's products or lowering costs per customer.

In the unsuccessful cases, IT was a peripheral activity or something new and not well understood by the industry (e.g., customer relationship software), and management was distracted by other issues.

Baumol (2002) notes that a fundamental empirical regularity of high-growth economies is a firm's use of innovation as a competitive weapon. In these economies, firms innovate to stay ahead or catch up to their competition. This is part of the "innovation machine" of the modern western economy. Our case studies suggest that IT fits this model of productivity growth: When IT is viewed and used as a competitive weapon and as central to the survival of the firm, it tends to enable the firm to increase productivity dramatically.

Potential Benefits of IT in Health

We now turn to the potential benefits of IT in health. What kind of productivity enhancement might be expected?

IT Productivity Enhancers

The six industries discussed above, all of which have high and growing IT investments, show a wide range in productivity improvements—from up to 18.9 percent per year (when combined with other elements), down to 0 percent per year. Furthermore, the six case studies establish the key IT productivity enhancers in the successful use of IT. These success factors are summarized in Table 4.2. We will use these factors to obtain a plausible productivity growth range for HIT. Because there are only six case studies to identify productivity enhancers, and we have not performed a detailed assessment or validation of the productivity enhancers, the following analysis in this section must be considered exploratory. One way to avoid

Table 4.2
Assessment of IT Productivity Enhancers in Healthcare

IT Productivity Enhancer	Healthcare Assessment
Raw growth in IT investment	Low to moderate—IT growth roughly one-third of high performing industries
Competition	Moderate—not as intense as retail or warehousing, for example; inefficiency not heavily punished
IT viewed as a competitive weapon	Not as of 2004, but inklings of change evident
Deregulation	No; trend toward increasing regulation; public suspicious of labor-saving moves
Opportunity for rapid technological improvement	Moderate; EHR will improve, but not at the rate of change found in telecoms, for example
Excessive merger activity	Probably not
Champion firm to drive change (e.g., Wal-Mart)	No
Integrated system—scope of organization conducive to optimized IT investment	No; significant network externalities; physicians and hospitals do not work together
Potential for HIT infrastructure to substitute for future labor or capital	Moderate

over-generalizing is to emphasize a range of possible healthcare IT productivity outcomes, which we will do at the end of this chapter.

The table outlines the strengths and weaknesses of the current healthcare system with respect to IT productivity enablers. Overall, the assessment is mixed at best. We consider each factor in turn then provide productivity scenarios based on the assessment.

Raw Growth of IT Investment. Although the microeconomic analysis clearly delineates the importance of complementary factors in extracting the value out of IT, the cases showed that the successful industries did invest a large and rapidly growing raw dollar amount in IT. Generally, in these industries, IT investment per employee ("IT capital intensity") grew faster than the national average and faster than it had historically. These industries increased their IT investment per year per employee at a rate in the mid-teens (see Table 4.3). In comparison, within healthcare, IT investment has a forecasted compounded annual growth rate (CAGR) from 1998–2006 of 8.4 percent,[9] and we estimate that it would be 1–2 percentage points less—perhaps 5–8 percent—if investment is calculated as investment per employee. There is not a noticeable investment uptick expected from 2004 to 2006.

---

[9] Sheldon Dorenfest and Associates (2004).

Table 4.3
IT Capital Intensity in Assorted Industries

Industry	IT Capital Intensity in 1999, $	Growth Rate 1995–1999, % (Using Available Data)
Telecommunications	265,000	17.3
Securities	16,000	17.2
Retail	1,900	18.9
Wholesale	18,500	16.9
Banking	27,200	16.8[a]
Hotels	2,311	11.0
U.S. average	9,130	13.9
Health	5,000–8,000[b] estimate	5-8 (1998-2006 estimate)

SOURCES: MGI, the Bureau of Labor Statistics, Dorenfest, and RAND analysis.
[a]After inflation.
[b]Assumes 25 percent depreciation of IT capital stock per year. Capital intensity is quite insensitive to changes in depreciation rate.

From our perspective, this less than stellar level of investment raises two concerns. First, the well documented fact that healthcare spends a lower percentage of its revenue on IT than other industries might suggest investment that is too low. Only the tech-light retail and hotel industries have lower capital intensity. Wholesale has three times the investment per employee. We find this argument only somewhat persuasive because interindustry comparisons of investment rates are very difficult to make. Second, and more serious, statistics show that HIT spending is not accelerating to any great degree, despite predictions of more rapid EHR uptake. As a percentage of healthcare revenue, HIT spending is virtually flat, and compared to other industries, its capital intensity growth rate is about one-third that of the high-performing industries. Because we are comparing growth rates, we do not have the interindustry comparison problem to the same degree; therefore, the comparison for HIT spending to IT spending in the high-productivity growth sectors should be judged appropriate. The comparison yields an unfavorable picture for the future of HIT-led productivity growth.

The capital intensity figures themselves show wide disparities between industries. IT capital in telecommunications includes the fiber and other telecommunications equipment, which explains its extraordinarily high capital intensity. Hotels and retail are more labor-intensive and less capital-intensive and have strong personal service orientations. Wholesale and banking are much higher than the average. These figures suggest that telecommunications and hotels are not as good comparators for health, because they are so different in their approaches to the use of IT. Healthcare is more like banking and wholesale, although hospitals have significant hotel-like functions. The figures also show that healthcare is below the national average, although not radically so.

IT Viewed as a Competitive Weapon. The level of competition in healthcare is a controversial subject and a detailed assessment is beyond the scope of this report. However, it seems safe to assert that compared to the level of competition in the "successful users" of IT or certainly in the "dramatic successes," there is less competition and certainly less-effective competition in healthcare, especially given the wave of provider mergers in the 1990s.

Among the successful users of IT, IT was considered a competitive weapon—a way to get ahead of competitors. This has not been the case to date for EHR.[10] Initially, EHR was adopted by academic centers interested in building knowledge and in pursuing other intrinsic motivations such as "it is part of our mission." However, this perception may be changing and policy could perhaps help this along, as we discuss in the next section. As of this writing, patients are beginning to show an interest in having their providers use EHR, and there is great interest on the part of government about how to pay for quality. Exactly how to operationalize paying for quality is not yet clear but is an area of active research.

Deregulation. There does not appear to be good news for IT productivity with respect to deregulation in healthcare. There is a trend toward more regulation, including legislating nurse staffing ratios. There may be important health reasons for the legislation; however, from the standpoint of trying to radically raise productivity through IT, the case studies suggest that this staffing ratio policy would hinder the transformation that IT could enable. IT tends to work as a complementary product that allows for radical redesign of work processes that entail changes in staffing, skill sets, and jobs. Regulation, especially labor regulation, might hinder these changes or stop them altogether.

Opportunity for Rapid Technological Improvement and Merger Activity. There is opportunity for technical improvement in EHR, as expressed by the gray literature and vendors, albeit less dramatic sheer technical improvement than the case for telecommunications. Merger activity is difficult to predict but should not be a greater impediment than it was to successful users.

Champion Firm. Healthcare does not have a champion firm to drive productivity, like Wal-Mart in big-box retail. Perhaps 15 years ago we would have argued that the staff model HMO would be the organization that is integrated and powerful enough to champion change. That is clearly not the case today and no substitute seems to be in sight. Instead, as yet unformed regional health initiative organizations (RHIOs) may be on the agenda to lead change.

---

[10] Although it has been for stand-alone revenue-enhancing IT innovations.

Lack of Organizational Integration. We turn now to some of the serious organizational issues with respect to capturing HIT value. Healthcare suffers, from an IT perspective, from a lack of organizational integration. There are significant network externalities in EHR. Physicians and hospitals do not work together and have not bought compatible EHR systems. Compare this state of affairs to, say, Wal-Mart, which as a single company simply dictates that its retail stores and its highly efficient warehouses have IT systems that can interoperate. In healthcare, it is as if the retail stores and the warehouses do not work together and do not particularly trust each other. Lack of interoperability is arguably the largest impediment to enhancing the value of HIT; our research repeatedly identified it as a barrier to successful adoption. Conceivably, privacy demands could forestall benefits of networked technology. These are discussed in other RAND work. However, the general conclusion is that privacy issues are manageable.

Potential for HIT Infrastructure to Substitute for Labor in the Future. Most successful IT-using industries were able to pay fixed costs on IT to enable future demand growth at low marginal cost, which in turn enables productivity growth. For example, telecommunications invested in mobile phone capacity, which allowed minutes to grow at low additional cost. It is not immediately apparent that such an economic transition could take place in healthcare. Healthcare has been very labor-intensive, and machines will not take care of large numbers of patients any time soon. It is possible that HIT could allow for much improved prevention, which would lead to higher quality at current funding and staffing levels. (For example, advanced monitoring of chronic conditions might promote longer lives at minimal cost.) It is much harder to see how HIT would wring out a large amount of labor from the current system, the way that online trading did in the securities trading industry.

Scenarios for Productivity Gains from HIT

From the above qualitative analysis, we generate scenarios for gains from HIT (see Figure 4.4). The "worst" case would be if expensive HIT, especially EHR, is purchased and then ignored and worked around, as providers become distracted by other matters and hospitals and physicians fail to solve the integration problem. If this happens, productivity improvements from HIT may be near zero, as in banking and hotels in the late 1990s.

The "excellent" case of 2 percent extra growth per year essentially replicates the success of the retail and wholesale sectors. This would indeed appear to be an excellent outcome for healthcare, and would be large enough to move the national productivity statistics in a positive direction as did retail and wholesale in the late 1990s. This size gain might not be likely, because the conditions in healthcare seem to be less favorable for IT-led productivity gains than they were in retail or wholesale in

Figure 4.4
Gains from HIT Improvement

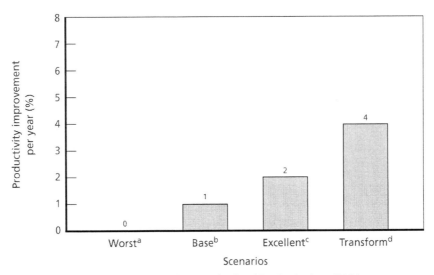

^aWorst: buy IT, get distracted, work around it (banking in the late 1990s).
^bBase: 1/2 of excellent (some competition, good attention to implementation).
^cExcellent: same as retail (deregulated, competitive).
^dTransform: fundamentally change the process of care (IT monitoring, integrated
  systems, personalized medicine, etc.).
RAND *MG272-4.4*

the late 1990s. IT investment is much lower, competition is not as intense, and there is no champion Wal-Mart-type firm to drive results. Also, if physicians and hospitals do not work together, it will hinder realizing the gains. This suggests that perhaps one-half of the full 2 percent gain might be a more realistic outcome, or even a moderately favorable outcome. Note that achieving this still requires attention to implementation (discussed above). The "Base" case of 1 percent is merely a subjective estimate. The reader may reasonably consider other projections as more likely, although projections of HIT productivity improvements of over 2 percent per year *given the current structure of U.S. healthcare* would appear to lack foundation. However, we include an upper estimate of 4 percent as a subjective upper bound.

When thought leaders talk about transforming healthcare with EHR and HIT in general, they are not talking about achieving roughly 1 percent productivity improvement per year. They are talking about the kinds of benefits seen in telecommunications or securities—IT-enabled gains of 8+ percent per year, year after year. These sectors show that it can be done. But they also show the ingredients needed to achieve this growth: intense competition, tremendous technical improvement, aggressive deregulation followed by minimal government intrusion except for anti-trust vigilance, firms that are integrated to the right level to make optimal IT investment decisions, and, finally, a physical ability to lay down a fixed IT investment and then have increased demand handled by the IT infrastructure rather than by more workers and more non-IT capital.

None of these conditions applies today in health, but these conditions suggest directions for policy improvements: Move healthcare toward the conditions proven in other industries to enhance IT and encourage raw investment in HIT.

Figure 4.5 shows the IT gains over 15 years from the different scenarios relative to the status quo. We chose 15 years because that provides enough time for savings to build, and there is evidence that at least one industry, telecommunications, was able to sustain productivity improvements over 15 years (and counting). The numbers above the bars are the percentage savings of the total healthcare spend of $37 trillion.[11] With a total 15-year healthcare spend of $37 trillion, the IT gains are very large, even though modest in percentage terms.

Under the "transform" scenario, savings are one-third of the healthcare budget on average. Under the base case, raw dollar savings are 9 percent. Comparing the

Figure 4.5
Potential 15-Year HIT Savings Are Large Because the Stakes Are Enormous

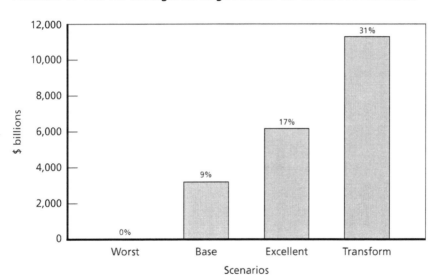

NOTE: See the note to Figure 4.4 for scenario definitions.
RAND *MG272-4.5*

---

[11] We assumed that the productivity increases decrease only cost, rather than increase quality. This is clearly counterfactual, but it allows for dollar quantification of the productivity benefits. Alternatively, one could assume that all benefits accrue to quality, or something in between. For example, if all benefits are in the form of increased quality, rather than costs, then under the base case QALYs (or some other measurement of quality) would improve $1 - 1/(1 - 0.09) = 10$ percent. This analysis makes no assumptions about to whom the savings accrue, although such an analysis was performed in the larger project.

worst case with the transformational case shows that IT savings can be from zero to a full one-third of the spending *depending on what else is going on in the industry.* This points out in another way how important other activities are and the extent that IT is a complementary good. IT is more effective when mixed with other ingredients and healthcare IT appears to be no exception.

What other ingredients should the government add to enable HIT led productivity growth, if any? We consider this question in the next section.

CHAPTER FIVE

Should the Government Intervene to Speed Diffusion of HIT?

To answer this question completely, policy analysis must quantify the costs and benefits of HIT,[1] forecast responses on the demand side and supply side of the market, and take into account the distortionary cost of raising a tax dollar.[2] Unfortunately, this is technically impossible because there is little recent empirically grounded research about how policy interventions change technology diffusion, let alone healthcare information technology diffusion. Some older sociological research from the 1970s details the failures of government mandates to change local practices, typically by failures of implementation (see Pressman and Wildavsky, 1984, for example).

Leaders in diffusion research agree that there is little evaluation of specific diffusion policies.[3] Stoneman and Diederen (1994), in *The Economic Journal*, state that it is surprising to find very few policy initiatives aimed at innovation diffusion.[4] Other leaders in the field, Tornatzky, Fleischer, et al. (1990, p. 239) state:

> In a study of over 200 published articles in the policy research and analysis field, over half the articles could best be described as based on "wisdom" or armchair theorizing. . . .

---

[1] Again, while our purview is HIT, the primary focus of the section will be on the crucial EHR technology.

[2] The welfare effects of speeding up adoption are complex and certainly not unambiguously positive (Stoneman and Diederen, 1994), not least because increased sales caused by faster adoption changes the time path of prices and quality in the industry via its effects on vendors. The medical community, however—at least those not charged directly with paying for systems—seems to have forged a consensus to push for faster adoption. This message comes from the IOM (1994) and the President's Information Technology Advisory Committee (PITAC) (2001), among others.

[3] One exception is Borzekowski (2002), who finds that state price regulation slowed adoption of IT in hospitals, whereas the Medicare prospective payment system increased speed of adoption.

[4] They go on to say: "For an evaluation of diffusion policy, one would wish to judge whether the costs incurred by government in pursuing a policy are greater or less than the welfare increases generated by the policy. There have been no evaluations of actual diffusion policies on those terms." p. 928. Karshenas and Stoneman in Stoneman (1995) state that we are currently very thin in policy analysis; the field is in its infancy.

Although this lack of empirical evidence is dismaying for a field that is almost 60 years old, there are some reasons for the dearth of hard data. It is very difficult to create the longitudinal datasets necessary to conduct policy analysis,[5] and there may be long latencies and many confounders in attempted empirical policy analyses. Therefore, we must proceed along theoretical lines and use caution in predicting the outcomes of specific policies.

This section addresses two basic questions:

1. In a reasonably competitive market such as the one for HIT, what is the rationale for *any* policy intervention? Why not just "let the market work?" That is often the least expensive option.
2. If there is a rationale for a policy intervention, what are the possible effects of the potentially beneficial intervention?

Rationales and Discussion of Government Intervention: Market Failure

We use fundamental economic welfare principles to evaluate normative rationales for policy intervention. The argument for speeding up adoption for any type of innovation must satisfy two conditions: (1) adoption is better than no adoption, and (2) adoption today is better than waiting and adopting tomorrow. In this framework, the basic reason for intervention is correcting a market failure.

There has been much discussion of the distorted incentives among patients, payers, and providers in healthcare. For example, patients do not pay on the margin anywhere near marginal cost of care; hospitals are often paid under fee-for-service, which rewards increased services rather than quality; physicians and hospitals work for different organizations, and incentives for quality are inadequate (too many medical errors) and yet also overdone in the name of quality (too many MRI machines and tests).

However, these distortions do not seem to provide adequate motivation by themselves for government intervention or subsidy. For example, why has HIT and especially expensive EHR diffused as widely as it has in the face of these distorted incentives? It is very important to identify which types of market failure appear to be the culprits in preventing HIT and specifically EHR from diffusing widely *and* deeply. We will attempt to do this below.

There are three general sources of potential market failure in HIT: imperfect information, including the key role of technical standards and quality measurement;

---

[5] We note that HIT has the same problem—any longitudinal datasets would have had to be created for this project specifically.

market power; and externalities. We cover each in turn and then discuss potential policies to address them.

Imperfect Information

In perfectly efficient markets, consumers costlessly collect full information about product price and quality. However, it is clear from our site visits and from the literature that hospitals acquire information incrementally through informal contact with their peers. These are discussed in the diffusion literature review above as epidemic effects via "activated peer group networks."

There are almost certainly epidemic effects ("peer group activation") in HIT, and we confirmed directly that HIT performance information flows between hospitals and from key medical opinion leaders to practicing physicians. Note that the "key opinion leader" terminology from medicine has very close cousins in social science terminology, with its "opinion leaders" who influence adoption behavior (Rogers, 1995). It is clear that opinion leaders drive adoption of innovations into the mainstream.

The academic literature identifies indirect evidence of epidemic effects in many other settings (see, for example, Kapur, 1995; Karshenas and Stoneman, 1993; and Czepiel, 1974).[6]

Epidemic effects in communication networks are important for policy because they could produce a multiplier effect with any policy-led increase in adoption. As a consequence, government intervention could induce a virtuous cycle, where adoption, either coerced or encouraged by incentives by the government, begets more adoption through peer-group recommendations. Government could augment adoption with ad campaigns or demonstration projects.

However, with hospital penetration of EHR nearing 25 percent in 2003 and increasing, the rationale for further demonstration programs diminishes. Virtually all providers are aware of EHR and know both the success and failure stories in its implementation. It is probably too late to consider demonstration programs in a broad

---

[6] Kapur (1995) finds epidemic effects in a theoretical diffusion framework. In this model, firms learn progressively through observing the experience of others. Given this prospect of social learning, every firm would prefer that other firms adopt before it does. (This is not a network externality because the firm benefits from the learning provided by the other firms' purchases rather than directly from the other firms' purchases.) Kapur finds that heterogeneity of firms is not essential to explain interfirm differences in adoption times. The model shows differences even among identical firms.

In the numerically controlled machine tool industry, the main factors affecting diffusion were found to be endogenous learning (epidemic effects), firm size, industry growth rates, the cost of the technology, and expected changes in the cost of the technology (Karshenas and Stoneman, 1993).

An early study describes epidemic effects in the continuous steel-casting industry (Czepiel, 1974). Using a directed-graph approach, the author identified informal communications networks and interactions within the industry. There was clear evidence that competing firms actively used friendship networks.

sense as a useful exercise although they might be useful if targeted on low-adopter populations.

A second source of imperfect information may be that expectations about future technological change are wrong. Incorrect expectations may lead to inefficient adoption decisions. However, correct expectations can lead to *less* socially optimal behavior. For example, suppose that the socially optimal diffusion path is faster than the one currently realized by providers. Further, suppose that providers erroneously believe that HIT prices will not fall. In this case, informing them of the true lower future prices may increase the delay in purchase, exacerbating the slow adoption problem.[7] Instead a commonly cited barrier was lack of evidence for return on investment.

Our site visits did not provide much evidence that providers have inaccurate expectations about future technological change. Undoubtedly, the world will unfold in unpredictable ways, but we found little evidence that decisionmakers had systematic misinformation.

Standards. It is well known that private markets may not by themselves efficiently choose a technical standard (the case of the VHS cassette is frequently cited in the literature). We found that some providers might be reluctant to invest in a technology that may be incompatible with emerging standards. They may delay HIT adoption because of uncertainty about its compatibility with the future community infrastructure. This compatibility and interoperability is valuable both within an organization as well as for sharing information between organizations. Standards are needed to make sure that similar functions are available in different EHR systems and that the format, structure, content, language, and transmission protocols are compatible between systems. Below, we will focus on this part of the standards issue. The issue in HIT with respect to standards is interoperability—different systems from different vendors must be able to talk to each other and share data to realize major gains for patient care.

For interoperability to be achieved, three things must be in order: (1) The separate pieces of hardware must be technically compatible, (2) software from different vendors must share a common medical vocabulary, and (3) the different systems must be electronically interfaced so that they can communicate with each other.

The first level of interoperability is largely in place. HL-7 provides a common machine language.

The second level is the focus of much of the current activity. The difficulty has been in finding standard medical terms. It has been difficult to find a standard medical language (Rector, 1999), partly because terminology changes over time. The

---

[7] We have asked hospitals about their price expectations. They do not expect prices to fall. They expect HIT quality to improve, but their own resources seem to be a larger factor in adoption than expectations of any major change in product variety or price.

World Health Organization produces a new International Classification of Diseases (ICD) every ten years or so. The switch from ICD-9 to ICD-10 is driving a 2004 overhaul of clinical terminology as well. Finally, a common patient identifier has not been agreed on.

The third level of interoperability has not been addressed to any significant degree. Analysts note that doing so would be very expensive with current hardware and software because the interface would have to be custom-made. Goldsmith (2003) believes that attempts to use the powerful new EHRs in the current fragmented information systems could result in huge waste and inefficiency. He suggests that the government specify minimum technical standards for clinical information systems.

It is important to point out that standardization would not eliminate competition in the software industry. Competition would continue, not only on price but on ease and speed of installation (a major factor mentioned in our site visits), speed of response, stability and reliability, user friendliness, and clinical decision support.

Although there is little empirical policy analysis about the effects of standards (Mowery, in Stoneman, 1995), we found a great deal of anecdotal evidence as well as studies described in the trade literature in healthcare and IT generally suggesting that standards are absolutely necessary to the smooth functioning of future EHR. The benefits of standardization appear to be well understood by the healthcare community. Comments from the thought leaders we interviewed largely echoed the National Committee on Vital and Health Statistics (NCVHS's) 2000 finding that "the greatest impediment to the adoption of healthcare information technology is the lack of complete and comprehensive standards for patient medical record information."

Moving data seamlessly between systems lies at the core of many quality and efficiency issues in healthcare (Brailer and Terasawa, 2003), and interoperability is at the heart of this ability. But the authors find low adoption rates for some of the standards that are critical to interoperability. For example, in the early 2000s, few providers implemented unique patient identifiers, interconnectivity, or standardized clinical terminology.

In summary, we found few detractors and many proponents of standards for EHR. The policy issue is what can be done and how quickly can it be done. Everyone wants standards, but any particular standard has detractors.

We surveyed evidence from other industries to understand how standards were applied and what contributed to their successful implementation. In the case of factory and office Local Area Networks, standardization depended on whether any firm was large enough to coordinate the entire market, be it General Motors (GM) as a buyer or IBM as a vendor (David and Greenstein, 1990, p. 20). In healthcare, no single provider is large enough to play a "GM" type of role, although the very largest employers could work together as buyers to impose standards.

However, the largest customer of healthcare in the United States is the federal government, and the largest government customer is the Centers for Medicare and

Medicaid Services (CMS). As the largest customer in healthcare, CMS could play a central role in driving standards.

In their analysis of seven case studies of standardization, Besen and Johnson (1986) identified several conditions that facilitated agreements on standards within voluntary organizations' committee process (i.e., not unlike healthcare standard-setting bodies). They found that (1) all major industry parties must be willing to participate; (2) any industry group has to overcome anti-trust objections; (3) a group must find a way to narrow choices, so that interested parties can more easily arrive at consensus; (4) groups must develop objective technical means for considering alternatives; and (5) there should be liberal licensing agreements and nominal royalty fees (quoted in David and Greenstein, 1990).

It appears that the HIT standards movement achieves most of these criteria, and the government could perhaps play the role of coordinator more ably than others. Indeed, CMS could address Besen and Johnson's five points above without having to play a role much different from its traditional one—including bringing industry parties together under the aegis of impartiality, dealing directly and authoritatively with antitrust issues, driving the group to narrow choices, and leaning on those with the "winning" standards to provide liberal licensing arrangements.

In summary, we found general consensus that standards are important and that government should play a role both in technical coordination and through its role as a major payer. Our analysis suggests that interoperability must be at the heart of future standardization efforts.

Inability to Measure Provider Quality Accurately. A pervasive problem in healthcare is the difficulty in measuring quality objectively. It is difficult to compete on what one cannot measure. In well-functioning markets, firms compete on quality, service, and price. In other industries studied in the previous chapter, it is taken for granted that quality benefits are noticed by the customers. For example, if Amazon.com invests in superior pick, pack, and ship IT that reduces shipping errors, there will be fewer customer complaints and returns. In healthcare, where quality is so important, providers instead compete more on price and service and provide little information on quality to the consumer or to employers. This is a fundamental and very serious market failure in healthcare. (For a recent article identifying this problem as central, see Porter and Teisberg, 2004.)

There is evidence that EHR may reduce this problem by allowing more sophisticated quality measurement tools, which generally require at least some data collection, manipulation, and computation, to be automated. By automating these quality measurement tools, they become much more usable.

Notice that in this area HIT could help and be helped in two ways. First, the inability to measure quality can conceivably retard the adoption of all quality-improving innovation, including HIT. This is the classic market failure problem: The market does not correctly value the quality-improving innovation. Second, HIT may have a somewhat unique ability to improve the measurement of quality in healthcare. Thus, adopting HIT may reduce the original market failure. There is a chicken-and-egg problem: HIT adoption is retarded by the market failure of inability to measure quality. But, to measure quality better, HIT must be adopted. Government may have a fairly strong rationale for intervening to lessen this problem. HIT not only improves quality, it improves the measurement of quality, which attacks the underlying market failure that is so pernicious in healthcare.

Government can intervene by promulgating HIT-enabled quality standards, paying for quality directly when it can measure it, and *possibly* subsidizing the purchase of EHR that enables better measurement of quality.

Market Power

Another general source of potential market failure can be market power. The economics literature identifies a number of market power rationales for intervention. Antitrust enforcement is a classic intervention to curtail excessive market power wielded by a firm. For example, it has been shown theoretically that diffusion may be too fast in unconcentrated markets because vendors compete with each other so vigorously that they essentially oversell the market.

The economics literature is split on whether concentrated industries (i.e., where providers have significant market power) produce more or less innovation. In summarizing much of this work, Mowery in Stoneman (1995) note that these studies generate no firm conclusion.[8]

Given these mixed results, the rationale for government intervention in HIT to correct for undue market power appears to be weak. There are neither empirical nor theoretical reasons to worry about too many or too few buyers or sellers in this market.[9] Although there are a substantial number of HIT suppliers—7 suppliers had 74 percent of the EHR market in 2002, with the remaining 26 percent composed of smaller players and self-developed systems—it seems implausible that they are overselling the market or need to be reined in by government. Thus, realigning market power does not appear to be a very credible reason for government intervention in HIT.

Related to issues of market power are potential supply-side policies involving changing incentives for vendors. They might include tax breaks, price subsidies, and, perhaps most prominently, standards-setting. Outside standards-setting, there appears to be little political interest in supply-side policies at this point because they clash overtly with the free-market policies of the United States. In addition, subsidies and tax breaks would partly create higher vendor profits and possibly higher prices

---

[8] See also Dearden, Ickes, and Samuelson (1990) and Levin et al. (1992).

[9] See Bhattacharya, Chatterjee, et al. (1986); Nault (1998), Nault et al. (1997), and Hoppe (2002) among others.

(although the effect is not clear-cut), neither result being a goal of policymakers or healthcare providers. Demand-side policies to assist providers who care directly for patients appear to be more likely policy options.

Externalities

A third potential source of market failure is externalities. Fundamentally, our respondents felt that the value of EHR is higher if others in the patient's care network already have it. This is a classic network externality. It can lead to a socially inefficient waiting game played by purchasers and to inefficiency in implementation.

Perhaps the most basic problem is that the hospital (the acute-care facility) rarely employs the physicians, who admit patients but conduct much of their care in remote locations. Further, pharmacies and labs have different ownership, partly because of well-intentioned conflict-of-interest regulations. These differences in ownership have come about for historical and probably understandable reasons, including preferred autonomy of physicians, patient choice, and some distrust between hospitals and physicians. But from the narrower perspective of maximizing HIT efficiency, the ownership differences are not optimal.

As an illustration of the difficulty, recall the retailing case study from the previous section and the benefits of IT in that setting. To make a comparison to healthcare, again imagine if Wal-Mart did not own its own warehouses, had low market share at those warehouses, and there was not a great deal of mutual trust between stores and warehouses. Such a situation would probably lead to less-than-optimal investment (lack of adoption) and to relatively poor implementation once the investment is made. This is the situation most of the time in healthcare.

It would be naïve to suggest reorganizing U.S. healthcare to optimize HIT decisions. Indeed, reorganizing options such as increasing vertical integration (that is, putting hospitals, doctors, labs, and pharmacies all under one organization) and accountability for a defined population might also be called a "staff HMO." This care model was the purported savior of U.S. healthcare in the early 1990s, but it was far from universally embraced by the customers. Furthermore, these disparate organizations would have greater incentive to work together if quality could be better measured. For example, New York State's publication of cardiac surgery mortality data led to big reductions in risk of surgery, despite the different players that needed to be brought to the table, as hospitals stopped some surgeons from operating or overhauled their failing departments. Nevertheless, the challenge for government is to craft a policy that reduces network externalities without requiring wholesale reorganization of the current system as an absolutely crucial piece of reform.[10]

---

[10] Although it is quite plausible, judging by other industries' histories, that a substantial reorganization will take place. The incentives should push organizations to move toward forms that can capture the benefits.

Reducing network externalities is a formidable challenge—as noted above, currently 83 percent of physician records are in paper form, so building interfaces from the hospital or other physicians' offices is technically impossible today (Goldsmith, 2003). Thus, the first step may be to digitize physician's offices. This may take policy initiatives, including possibly subsidies, since individual offices are generally capital-poor. The rationale is that network externalities constitute a market failure, preventing most of the gains of the IT investment from accruing to the physician that needs to make the investment.

Transfers among parties (rather than outright government payments) are the usual economic prescription for reducing network problems. For example, a hospital that installs EHR first could pay physicians' offices to join its network. At least theoretically, this arrangement reduces the problem, because it gets all the parties to act more on the collective EHR benefit (since they now formally share the benefits).[11] There are two problems with transfers in this context: (1) They are illegal in healthcare under some circumstances, and (2) they are certain to be expensive to implement and that money will have to come from somewhere. Direct payments from hospitals to physicians have been illegal under the Stark laws, and it might be difficult to separate EHR payments from (illegal) payments for referrals. Even if these problems can be overcome, implementing these payments can be daunting. Establishing regional health information organizations, likely enablers of transfer payments, may costs millions per city (or similar unit) and take two years to implement.

The standards problem and the network externalities problem combine into one overarching problem: The EHR systems must be able to communicate with each other and the healthcare providers must have the incentive (not currently provided by the imperfect market) to adopt and use the technology. This problem could be addressed by promoting "community connectivity," which has been receiving increased attention. Furthermore, it is recognized that there is no management across many boundaries (e.g., hospital/physician practice) and policy must take this into account. In other words, this concept partly aims to correct some of the market and organizational failures of healthcare IT and, in a broad sense, this analysis strongly supports those efforts.

An intervention to address network externalities may be led by both federal and state governments. However, the policy needs to encourage linking the local providers for any specific patient or at least remove current impediments to those linkages. To assist with this, the government may need to consider relaxing inurement of

---

[11] In fact, under not implausible modeling assumptions, allowing transfers may provide correct incentives to achieve socially optimal adoption times. In other words, at least theoretically, subsidies may not be necessary; allowing transfers may suffice (the author's microeconomic analysis is available on request).

benefit regulations with respect to HIT.[12] Such changes are naturally very complex and need to be carefully considered before implementation.

It has been noted by some in the trade literature that there is a "problem" because not all of the beneficiaries of HIT, such as insurers and patients, pay for HIT directly. Usually, only the provider pays for HIT. However, the existence of a group that benefits but does not pay directly is *not* a sufficient reason for market intervention. For example, consumers do not pay cereal companies for IT upgrades to make better cereal. In that market, consumers prefer low-cost, high-quality cereals and the cereal companies decide if IT will help them meet those preferences and invest accordingly.

It can be a poor idea to appeal for subsidies on the basis of "shared cost for shared benefit," because in efficiently functioning markets, costs are rarely shared. In a market with poor information, such as quality measurement in healthcare, HIT could improve quality indirectly by improving measurement of quality. But then the reason for the intervention is improving quality measurement, not that the customers need to pay for the improvement per se. Instead, firms must decide whether IT is a useful competitive weapon and then invest and use it effectively to profit. A tax or mandate on insurers to pay for HIT, for example, flies in the face of this logic and could possibly blunt instead of sharpen the weapon of HIT as a means of succeeding in the healthcare marketplace.

Summary of Key Findings and Concluding Observations

EHR has diffused to up to 32 percent of the acute-care hospital population after a 20+ year latency. It is diffusing at a rate consistent with other similar information technologies characterized by network externalities and high complexity. HIT works by enabling improvements in work processes. It may or may not be the prime mover of improvements. Because of its complementary role, benefits of IT vary widely across industries and regulatory environments. HIT is possibly delivering incremental labor productivity benefits of 1 percent per year; the range may be from 0 percent to perhaps 4 percent per year. With the base case improvement of 1 percent per year, the savings are in the range of $3 trillion dollars over 15 years.

Extraordinarily effective implementation within the *current* healthcare system might double this number, in which case healthcare would be using IT as effectively as the highly efficient retail and wholesale sectors used IT in the late 1990s. Other industries have undergone productivity transformations of 8 percent per year or more, enabled by the combination of deregulation, competition, and rapid improvement in IT. Transformational productivity improvements, seen in telecommu-

---

[12] Inurement of benefit refers to the federal prohibition against hospitals' compensating physicians for referrals.

nications and securities trading, are out of reach given healthcare's structure and dependence on labor and constant capital deepening. However, if such transformations were achieved, they could lower healthcare costs per unit of quality by 75 percent after 15 years. This is well worth the investment to society, but how much should the government, or other agencies responsible for policy, help the private market to achieve these gains?

A number of attractive policy avenues deserve further study. The policy avenues discussed below are active priorities among the many policymaking stakeholders.[13] The purpose of this report has been to provide a better conceptual and empirical basis for pursuing certain general lines of policy, rather than to discuss specific current proposals in much depth (which are better addressed in a series of ongoing issue papers, for example, than in full reports). Note also that the list below is still very broad. The question may be asked: Ultimately, is HIT not a narrower concern within healthcare, albeit an important one? There are at least two reasons for the broad list below. First, HIT and especially EHR is a technology that affects virtually all players in the healthcare community. It is a broad technology and requires a broad policy to be effective.

Second, the value of HIT is maximized when complementary investments are made. The value of HIT swings widely depending on what else is going on in the system. In healthcare, there is a lot going on, much of it unhelpful to maximizing the HIT investment. Accordingly, the policy remit to optimize HIT efficiency touches on a number of healthcare problems, many all too familiar to health policymakers.

This report's research lends support to developing policy and solutions in the following policy areas:

Coordinate Standards Immediately

It is important to continue to coordinate standards and push for initiatives that improve the chances for interoperability, especially within regional communities. Standards should be improved without affecting competition among competing EHR vendors.

Work to Improve Quality Measurement

The benefits of improving quality measurement are twofold: First, improving quality measurement will help to overcome the market failure of not recognizing quality, which will spur the adoption of quality-improving innovation, including HIT. Second, there is a feedback loop: Adoption itself will reduce this market failure, because EHR holds the promise of improving quality measurement, largely by automating an otherwise dauntingly labor-intensive process of quality management. Some have ar-

---

[13] A forthcoming report will give a more detailed review of current policy efforts, which are very numerous.

gued that this difficulty in measuring and competing on quality is the most important problem in healthcare.

In addition to these two strong rationales for policy in this area, there is still a
third: The government, as a key customer, has the opportunity to improve providers'
performance. A strong series of results in the theory of innovation show that a "smart
buyer" can drive an industry to higher efficiency. (For example, consider the effects
of Japanese consumers' cutting-edge tastes on Japanese consumer electronics firms.)
To date, the government as a healthcare buyer has done much to affect the system
but much less to reform the system. HIT can help transform the system and help
government push through complementary changes in quality measurement and pay
for performance that should improve the system. Perhaps this is the area that holds
out the greatest promise for truly transformative HIT-enabled change.

The government should consider what quality-based rewards it could use to virtually require that providers pursue EHR. Is there something the government can do
without blatantly interfering with private economic transactions to assist with this
goal?

Reduce Network Externalities

The government can work to lessen network externalities, which should lead to more
adoption of EHR and especially more effective adoption. Our analysis suggests that
the federal government could lead an intervention, but a successful policy needs to
encourage linking the local providers for any specific patient. To assist with these efforts, the government may need to consider further relaxing inurement of benefit
regulations with respect to HIT. Because of network externalities, some selective
grants or subsidies *may* be optimal for underfunded physicians' offices, but we do not
view this as proven. Alternatively, allowing transfer payments (connect fees or bonuses) among members of the regional network may be a good idea (and less expensive for the government), if legal issues can be overcome. The allowed financial incentives should be targeted at improving community connectivity directly (e.g., IT
hardware), or indirectly (e.g., digitizing patient paper records).

However, there needs to be further, detailed research at the firm and regional
level to guide policy here. This report identifies a promising research agenda but
must stop short of detailed recommendations; it certainly does not endorse subsidies
at this time.

Recognize That HIT Requires Complementary Investments

It has been shown in other industries that IT is much more effective when combined
with vigorous competition and deregulation. Complex IT such as EHR is definitely
not a stand-alone or plug-and-play type of benefit. Rather, it can, if (and only if)
used appropriately, deliver dramatic changes in the overall delivery of care that could
radically improve quality and lower the cost of delivering that higher quality.

The reverse side of this observation is that preventing complementary changes in work processes by stifling competition or direct regulation might stop HIT gains outright. For example, HIT efficiencies conceivably allow reductions in nurse staffing. Realizing those reductions would be greatly hindered in California, where floor staffing ratios are fixed by state law. Therefore, the indirect benefits of allowing competition and reorganization should be considered along with any direct benefits of labor market or, more generally, input to production regulation.

Make Policy Decisions That Turn HIT into a Competitive Weapon

Industrial history shows that IT is most efficiently used when used as a competitive weapon central to a firm's business. This result is highly consistent with a more general theory of successful innovation in a modern economy. In the context of health policy, one way to sharpen the competitive advantage of IT might be to reimburse quality in Medicare more directly, where measuring quality is possible only with an EHR-enabled quality tracking system. Another fruitful line of research would be to study whether Medicare should pay for EHR-enabled claims. In such a world, providers improve profitability by using EHR and using it well and having the credible quality measures to prove that they are using it well. (Note that this policy prescription is related to the quality-measurement policies above, because they both address the fundamental market failure of poorly measured quality.)

Before the government can implement such efforts, however, it needs to determine lead time to install EHR widely and deeply, to determine how to pay for quality and not just the physical presence of an EHR, to calculate the correct size of the premium for IT-submitted claims, and finally, to quantify and address the size of any unfunded mandate. To encourage broad use within a network, payment should be structured to reward very broad physician participation rather than simply the presence of some kind of EHR in the provider.

Discuss and Agree Whether 100 Percent EHR Penetration Is a Societal Goal, Because History Suggests That It Will Not Happen Without Intervention

EHR diffusion has reached more than 20 percent of acute-care hospitals and may soon go over 50 percent. However, the analysis in Chapter Two suggests, based on review of other IT innovations, that penetration will not reach 100 percent of the provider community. If 100 percent EHR is a societal goal, because society wishes to maximize network gains or avoid a two-tier system, or both, then some form of subsidy for the more disadvantaged and isolated practices is likely necessary. The issues for these offices should likely be interoperability and community connectivity to maximize gains from HIT and EHR in particular.

Adopt an Incremental, Evolutionary Perspective on Policy Development

There are few more important areas for proper government economic policy than healthcare, specifically HIT. It is only a slight overstatement to say that future U.S. competitiveness and the health of its citizens depend upon it.

Given the enormous stakes, the uncertainty in the effects of policy, and the latency of the gains from HIT implementation, it might be wise to heed organizational theorists' views on evolutionary policy analysis. Evolutionary theory of organizations and policy suggests that policymakers have bounded rationality, just like firms (or providers).[14] Although policymakers do not know the effects of policy with much certainty, they have superior ability to coordinate across groups and a rationale to fix market failures. Evolutionary theorists, as well as some business school academics, suggest that it is usually best to be able to evaluate policies and business strategies early and adapt quickly.[15] Such a perspective is almost certainly wise in this context.

This suggests incremental government interventions with rapid review of results, with follow-on funding for successful interventions. This will help to avoid mistakes and allows policy a better chance to keep up with the rapid technical change in IT and in healthcare organization.

---

[14] Metcalfe (1994, 1995, p. 418).

[15] Metcalfe (1994), Christensen et al. (2000), and Christensen and Raynor (2003).

Bibliography

Anderson, J. G., and S. J. Jay, "Computers and Clinical Judgment: The Role of Physician Networks," *Social Science & Medicine*, Vol. 20, No. 10, 1985, pp. 969–979.

Anderson, R. L., and D. J. Ortinau, "Exploring Consumers' Postadoption Attitudes and Use Behaviors in Monitoring the Diffusion of a Technology-Based Discontinuous Innovation," *Journal of Business Research*, Vol. 3, No. 17, 1988, pp. 283–298.

Ash, J., P. Gorman, V. Seshadri, and W. Hersh, "Computerized Physician Order Entry in U.S. Hospitals: Results of a 2002 Survey," *Journal of the American Medical Association*, Vol. 11, No. 2, 2004, pp. 95–99.

"Automation of Web Logistics Can Reduce Return Processing Costs," *Direct Marketing*, Vol. 65, No. 4, 2001.

Axam, R., and D. Jerome, "A Guide to ERP Success," *The Project Office, Teams, Processes and Tools.*

Baily, M. N., "Distinguished Lecture on Economics in Government, The New Economy: Post Mortem or Second Wind?" *Journal of Economic Perspectives*, Vol. 16, No. 2, 2002, pp. 3–22.

Baldwin, F. D., "CPRs in the Winner's Circle," *Healthcare Informatics*, 2003.

Basu, S., J. G. Fernald, N. Oulton, and S. Srinivasan, "The Case of the Missing Productivity Growth: Or, Does Information Technology Explain Why Productivity Accelerated in the United States But Not the United Kingdom?" Cambridge, Mass.: National Bureau of Economic Research, working paper #10010, 2003.

Batiz-Lazo, B., and D. Wood, "Information Technology Innovations and Commercial Banking: A Review and Appraisal from an Historical Perspective," *Economic History*, Economics Working Paper Archive, WUSTL, #0211001, 2002.

Baumol, W. J., *The Free-Market Innovation Machine*, Princeton, N.J.: Princeton University Press, 2002.

Baur, C., "Limiting Factors on the Transformative Powers of E-Mail in Patient-Physician Relationships: A Critical Analysis," *Health Communication*, Vol. 12, No. 3, 2000, pp. 239–259.

Besen, S. M., and L. L. Johnson, *Compatibility Standards, Competition and Innovation in the Broadcasting Industry*, Santa Monica, Calif.: RAND Corporation, R-3453-NSF, 1986.

Bhattacharya, S., K. Chatterjee, et al., "Sequential Research and the Adoption of Innovations," *Oxford Economic Papers*, Vol. 38, No. 0, 1986, pp. 219–243.

Bikson, T. K., *Understanding the Implementation of Office Technology*, Santa Monica, Calif.: RAND Corporation, N-2619-NSF, 1987.

Bikson, T. K., *Organizational Trends and Electronic Media: Work in Progress*, Santa Monica, Calif.: RAND Corporation, RP-307, 1997.

Bikson, T. K., S. A. Law, M. Markovich, and B. T. Harder, *Facilitating the Implementation of Research Findings: Review, Synthesis, Recommendations*, Santa Monica, Calif.: RAND Corporation, RP-481, 1995.

Bikson, T. K., S. A. Law, M. Markovich, and B. T. Harder, *Facilitating the Implementation of Research Findings: A Summary Report*, Santa Monica, Calif.: RAND Corporation, RP-595, 1997.

Blair, J., "The Electronic Health Record Today," *Healthcare Informatics*, 2003.

Blume, S., "Early Warning in the Light of Theories of Technological Change," *International Journal of Technology Assessment in Health Care*, Vol. 14, No. 4, 1998, pp. 613–623.

Borzekowski, R., "Measuring the Cost Impact of Hospital Information Systems: 1987–1994," 2002.

Borzekowski, R., "Healthcare Finance and the Early Adoption of Hospital Information Systems," Board of Governors of the Federal Reserve System, 2002, pp. 1–32.

Brailer, D. J., and E. L. Terasawa, "Use and Adoption of Computer-based Patient Records," Prepared for California HealthCare Foundation, 2003, available at www.chcf.org.

Burke, D. E., B. B. Wang, et al., "Exploring Hospitals' Adoption of Information Technology," *Journal of Medical Systems*, Vol. 26, No. 4, 2002, pp. 349–355.

Chatfield, A. T., and P. Yetton, "Strategic Payoff from EDI as a Function of EDI Embeddedness," *Journal of Management Information Systems*, Vol. 16, No. 4, 2000, pp. 195–224.

Chatterjee, R., and J. Eliashberg, "The Innovation Diffusion Process in a Heterogeneous Population: A Micromodeling Approach," *Management Science*, Vol. 36, No. 9, 1990, pp. 1057–1079.

Chattoe, E., and N. Gilbert, *A Basic Simulation of Information Diffusion*, Centre for Research on Simulation in the Social Sciences (CRESS), Guildford, United Kingdom: Department of Sociology, University of Surrey, 1998.

Chau, P.Y.K., and K. Y. Tam, "Organizational Adoption of Open Systems: A 'Technology-Push, Need Push' Perspective," *Information & Management*, Vol. 37, No. 5, 2000, pp. 229–239.

Chiasson, M. W., and C. Y. Lovato "The Health Planning Context and Its Effect on a User's Perceptions of Software Usefulness," *Canadian Journal of Public Health*, Vol. 91, No. 3, 2000, pp. 225–258.

Christensen, C. M., R. Bohmer, et al., "Will Disruptive Innovations Cure Healthcare?" *Harvard Business Review*, Vol. 78, No. 5, 2000, p. 102.

Christensen, C. M., and M. E. Raynor, *The Innovator's Solution,* Boston, Mass.: Harvard Business School Press, 2003.

Colombo, M. G., and R. Mosconi, "Complementarity and Cumulative Learning Effects in the Early Diffusion of Multiple Technologies," *Journal of Industrial Economics*, Vol. 43, No. 1, 1995, pp. 13–48.

Czepiel, J. A., "Word-of-Mouth Processes in the Diffusion of a Major Technological Innovation," *Journal of Marketing Research*, Vol. 11, No. 2, 1974, pp. 172–180.

Dansky, K. H., L. D. Gamm, et al., "Electronic Medical Records: Are Physicians Ready?" *Journal of Health Care Management,* Vol. 44, No. 6, 1999, pp. 440–454; discussion 454-5.

David, P., and S. Greenstein, "The Economics of Compatibility Standards: An Introduction to Recent Research," *Economics of Innovation and New Technology,* Vol 1, 1990, pp. 3–41.

Dearden, J., B. W. Ickes, and L. Samuelson, "To Innovate Or Not to Innovate: Incentives and Innovation in Hierarchies," *The American Economic Review,* Vol. 80, No. 5, 1990, pp. 1105–1124.

Detmer, D. E., "Information Technology for Quality Healthcare: A Summary of United Kingdom and United States Experiences," *Quality Healthcare,* Vol. 9, No. 3, 2000, pp. 181–189.

Dong, D., and A. Saha, "He Came, He Saw, (and) He Waited: An Empirical Analysis of Inertia in Technology Adoption," *Applied Economics*, Vol. 30, No. 7, 1998, pp. 893–905.

Dorenfest, S., HIMSS Analytics Database (formerly the Dorenfest IHDS+ Database).

Drazen, E., and J. Fortin, "Digital Hospitals Move Off the Drawing Board," Prepared for California HealthCare Foundation, 2003.

Eger, M. S., R. L. Godkin, and S. R. Valentine, "Physicians' Adoption of Information Technology: A Consumer Behavior Approach," *Health Mark Q*, Vol. 19, No. 2, 2001, pp. 3–21.

England, I., D. Stewart, and S. Walker, "Information Technology Adoption in Healthcare: When Organisations and Technology Collide," *Australian Health Review*, Vol. 23, No. 3, 2000, pp. 176–185.

Frewer, L., "Risk Perception, Social Trust, and Public Participation in Strategic Decision Making: Implications for Emerging Technologies," *Ambio*, Vol. 28, No. 61999, pp. 569–574.

Geroski, P. A., "Models of Technology Diffusion," CEPR Discussion Paper No. 2146, 1999.

Geroski, P. A., "Models of Technology Diffusion," *Research Policy*, Vol. 29, Nos. 4–5, 2000, pp. 603–625.

Goldsmith, J., *Digital Medicine: Implications for Healthcare Leaders*, Chicago, Ill.: Health Administration Press, 2003.

Goldsmith, J., D. Blumenthal, et al., "Federal Health Information Policy: A Case of Arrested Development," *Health Affairs* (Millwood), Vol. 22, No. 4, 2003, pp. 44–55.

Gordon, R. J., "Comments and Discussions," *Brookings Papers on Economic Activity*, Vol. 2, 2002, pp. 245–265.

Gowrisankaran, G., and J. Stavins, "Network Externalities and Technology Adoption: Lessons from Electronic Payments," Cambridge, Mass.: National Bureau of Economic Research, working paper #8943, May 2002.

Grover, V., K. Fiedler, et al., "Empirical Evidence on Swanson's Tri-Core Model of Information Systems Innovation," *Information Systems Research*, Vol. 8, No. 3, 1997, pp. 273–287.

Gust, C., and J. Marquez, "International Comparisons of Productivity Growth: Recent Developments," *Business Economics*, 2001, pp. 55–62.

Hagland, M., "Doctors' Orders," *Healthcare Informatics*, 2003.

Hagland, M., "Emerging Picture Shows Technical Integration and Business Consolidation," *Healthcare Informatics*, 2003.

Hall, B. H., and B. Khan, "Adoption of New Technology," Cambridge, Mass.: National Bureau of Economic Research, working paper #9730, May 2003.

HIMSS Healthcare CIO Survey, 2003.

"Hooker Furniture Sees the Benefits of Real-Time Information Visibility—Wireless Distribution and Shipping Systems Raise Productivity 20% and May Eliminate Need to Take Inventory," *Frontline Solutions*, January 2000.

Hoppe, H. C., "The Timing of New Technology Adoption: Theoretical Models and Empirical Evidence," *Manchester School*, Vol. 70, No. 1, 2002, pp. 56–76.

Hornstein, A., and P. Krusell, "The IT Revolution: Is It Evident in the Productivity Numbers?" *Federal Reserve Bank of Richmond Economic Quarterly*, Vol. 86, No. 4, 2000, pp. 49–78.

Hu, P. J.-H., P.Y.K. Chau, and O.R.L. Sheng, *Investigation of Factors Affecting Healthcare Organizations' Adoption of Telemedicine Technology*, 33rd Hawaii International Conference on System Sciences, Maui, Hawaii, 2000.

IOM, *Adopting New Medical Technology*, Washington, D.C.: National Academy Press, 1994.

Jardini, D., "From Iron to Steel: The Recasting of the Jones and Laughlin Workforce between 1885 and 1896," *Technology and Culture*, Vol. 35, 1995, pp. 271–301.

Jorgenson, D. W., and K. J. Stiroh, "Information Technology and Growth," *American Economic Review*, Vol. 89, No. 2, 1999, pp. 109–115.

Kapur, S., "Technological Diffusion with Social Learning," *The Journal of Industrial Economics*, Vol. 43, No. 2, 1995, pp. 173–195.

Karshenas, M., and P. L. Stoneman, "Rank, Stock, Order, and Epidemic Effects in the Diffusion of New Process Technologies: An Empirical Model," *The Rand Journal of Economics*, Vol. 24, No. 4, 1993, pp. 503–528.

Karshenas, M., and P. L. Stoneman, "Techological Diffusion," in P. L. Stoneman, ed., *Handbook of the Economics of Innovation and Technological Change*, United Kingdom: Blackwell, 1995, pp. 265–297.

Katz, M. L., and C. Shapiro, "Technology Adoption in the Presence of Network Externalities," *Journal of Political Economy*, Vol. 94, No. 4, 1986, pp. 822–841.

Kuan, K.K.Y., and P.Y.K. Chau, "A Perception-Based Model for EDI Adoption in Small Businesses Using a Technology-Organization-Environment Framework," *Information & Management*, Vol. 38, No. 8, 2001, pp. 507–521.

Lai, V. S., and J. L. Guynes, "An Assessment of the Influence of Organizational Characteristics on Information Technology Adoption Decision: A Discriminative Approach," *IEEE Transactions on Engineering Management*, Vol. 44, 1997, pp. 146–157.

Larsen, T. J., and E. McGuire, eds., *Information Systems Innovation and Diffusion: Issues and Directions*, Hershey, Penn.: Idea Group Publishing, 1998.

Levin, S. G., S. L. Levin, et al., "Market Structure, Uncertainty, and Intrafirm Diffusion: The Case of Optical Scanners in Grocery Stores," *The Review of Economics and Statistics*, Vol. 74, No. 2, 1992, pp. 345–350.

Liberatore, M. J., and D. Breem, "Adoption and Implementation of Digital-Imaging Technology in the Banking and Insurance Industries," *IEEE Transactions on Engineering Management*, Vol. 44, 1997, pp. 367–377.

Loh, L., and N. Venkatraman, "Diffusion of Information Technology Outsourcing: Influence Sources and the Kodak Effect," *Information Systems Research*, Vol. 3, No. 4, 2001, pp. 334–358.

Majumdar, S., and S. Venkataraman, "Network Effects and the Adoption of New Technology: Evidence from the U.S. Telecommunications Industry," *Strategic Management Journal*, Vol. 19, 1998, pp. 1045–1062.

Mansfield, E., "Technical Change and the Rate of Imitation," *Econometrica: Journal of the Econometric Society*, Vol. 29, No. 4, 1961, pp. 741–766.

Marhula, D. C., "Is e-Health FACT or FICTION," *Healthcare Informatics*, 2003.

McKinsey Global Institute, *U.S. Productivity Growth 1995–2000, Understanding the Contribution of Information Technology Relative to Other Factors*, Washington, D.C., 2001.

Medical Records Institute, *4th Annual Survey of Electronic Health Record Trends and Usage,* sponsored by SNOMED, 2001.

Metcalfe, J. S., "Evolutionary Economics and Technology Policy," *The Economic Journal,* Vol. 104, No. 425, 1994, pp. 931–944.

Metcalfe, S., "The Economic Foundations of Technology Policy: Equilibriumand Evolutionary Perspectives," in P. Stoneman, ed., *Handbook of the Economics of Innovation and Technological Change,* United Kingdom: Blackwell, 1995.

Metzger, J., and F. Turisco, "Computerized Physician Order Entry: A Look at the Vendor Marketplace and Getting Started," First Consulting Group, 2001.

Miller, R. H., and I. Sim, "Physicians' Use of Electronic Medical Records: Barriers and Solutions," *Pursuit of Quality,* 2004, pp. 116–126.

Miller, R. H., I. Sim, and J. Newman, "Electronic Medical Records: Lessons from Small Physician Practices," prepared for California HealthCare Foundation, Oakland, Calif., 2003.

Mitropoulos, P., and C. B. Tatum, "Technology Adoption Decisions in Construction Organizations," *Journal of Construction Engineering and Management,* Vol. 125, No. 5, 1999, pp. 330–338.

Modern Physician/Price Waterhouse Coopers survey, administered online at *Modern Physician* website, 2003.

Moore, G. C., and I. Benbasat, "Development of an Instrument to Measure the Perceptions of Adopting an Information Technology Innovation," *Information Systems Research,* Vol. 2, No. 3, 1991, pp. 192–222.

Moore, J., Jr., "Barriers to Technology Adoption," *Environmental Science & Technology,* Vol. 28, 1994, pp. 193A–195A.

Mowery, D., "The Practice of Technology Policy," in Stoneman, P., ed., *Handbook of the Economics of Innovation and Technological Change,* United Kingdom: Blackwell, 1995.

National Health Expenditure Statistics, available at www.nhe.gov.

Nault, B. R., "Information Technology and Organizational Design: Locating Decisions and Information," *Management Science,* Vol. 44, No. 10, 1998, pp. 1321–1335.

Nault, B. R., R. A. Wolfe, et al., "Support Strategies to Foster Adoption of Interorganizational Innovations," *IEEE Transactions on Engineering Management,* Vol. 44, 1997, pp. 378–389.

Nordhaus, W. D., "Productivity Growth and the New Economy," *Brookings Papers on Economic Activity,* Vol. 2, 2002, pp. 211–244.

O'Callaghan, R., "Technology Diffusion and Organizational Transformation: An Integrative Framework," in T. Larsen, and E. McGuire, eds., *Information Systems Innovation and Diffusion: Issues and Directions,* Hersehy, Pa.: Idea Group Publishing, 1998.

Oliner, S., and D. Sichel, "The Resurgence of Growth in the Late 1990s: Is Information Technology the Story?" *Journal of Economic Perspectives*, Vol. 14, No. 4, 2000, pp. 3–22.

Ortiz, E., "Federal Initiatives," *Healthcare Informatics*, 2003.

Pathak, G., and S. K. Goyal, "Transforming Business Through Information Technology," *Computer*, 1999, pp. 40–41.

Perrotta, P., "EDI Lowers Transaction Costs for Texas Grocer," Supermarketnews.com, 2002, pp. 19, 21.

Pilat, D., "Digital Economy Going for Growth," *Observer*, Vol. 237, 2003, pp. 15–17.

Porter, M. E., and E. O. Teisberg, "Redefining Competition in Healthcare," *Harvard Business Review*, June 2004.

Powell, W. W., and P. J. DiMaggio, eds., *The New Institutionalism in Organizational Analysis*, Chicago, Ill.: University of Chicago Press, 1991.

Prater, E., and M. Sobol, *A Financial Tool for Assessing Comparative Cost Savings and Profitability of Information Technology Investment in HMOs,* paper presented at the Decision Sciences Institute Southwest Region Conference, San Antonio, Texas, 2003.

President's Information Technology Advisory Committee, "Transforming Health Care Through Information Technologies," 2001.

Pressman, J., and A. Wildavsky, *Implementation: How Great Expectations in Washington are Dashed in Oakland,* Berkeley, Calif.: University of California Press, 1984.

Queree, A., "Portal Power," *Global Finance*, Vol. 14, No. 4, 2000, pp. 65–66.

Raghupathi, W., and J. Tan, "Strategic Uses of Information Technology in Healthcare: A State-of-the-Art Survey," *Topics in Health Information Management*, Vol. 20, No. 1, 1999, pp. 1–15.

Rai, A., T. Ravichandran, et al., "How to Anticipate the Internet's Global Diffusion," *Communications of the ACM,* Vol. 41, No. 10, 1998, pp. 97–106.

Raman, A., N. DeHoratius, and Z. Ton, "Execution: The Missing Link in Retail Operations," *California Management Review*, Vol. 43, No. 3, 2001, pp. 136–152.

Rector, A., "Clinical Terminology: Why Is It So Hard?" *Methods of Information in Medicine,* Vol. 38, No. 4, 1999, pp. 239–252.

Ricci, R. J., "The Internet as a Computer," *Healthcare Informatics*, 2003.

Robison, K. K., and E. M. Crenshaw, "Post-Industrial Transformations and Cyber-Space: A Cross-National Analysis of Internet Development," *Social Science Research,* Vol. 32, No. 3, 2003, pp. 519–524.

Rogers, E. M., *Diffusion of Innovations,* 4th ed., New York: Free Press, 1995.

Romeo, A. A., "Interindustry and Interfirm Differences in the Rate of Diffusion of an Innovation," *Review of Economics and Statistics,* Vol. 57, No. 3, 1975, pp. 311–319.

Rosenau, P. V., "Managing Medical Technology: Lessons for the United States from Quebec and France," *International Journal of Health Services*, Vol. 30, No. 3, 2000, pp. 617–639.

Saloner, G., and A. Shepard, "Adoption of Technologies with Network Effects: An Empirical Examination of the Adoption of Automated Teller Machines," *The Rand Journal of Economics*, Vol. 26, No. 3, 1995, pp. 479–501.

Santhanam, R., and E. Hartono, "Issues in Linking Information Technology Capability to Firm Performance," *MIS Quarterly*, Vol. 27, No. 1, 2003, pp. 125–153.

Silverberg, G., G. Dosi, and L. Orsenigo, "Innovation, Diversity and Diffusion: A Self-Organisation Model," *The Economic Journal*, Vol. 98, No. 393, 1988, pp. 1032–1054.

Southon, G., C. Sauer, et al., "Lessons from a Failed Information Systems Initiative: Issues for Complex Organisations," *International Journal of Medical Informatics*, Vol. 55, No. 1, 1999, pp. 33–46.

Standish Group Report, "Chaos," T23E-T10E, West Yarmouth, Mass., 1995.

Stiroh, K. J., "Information Technology and the U.S. Productivity Revival: What Do the Industry Data Say?" *American Economic Review*, Vol. 92, No. 5, 2002, pp. 1559–1576.

Stoneman, P., and M-J Kwon, "The Diffusion of Multiple Process Technologies," *The Economic Journal*, Vol. 104, No. 423, 1994, pp. 420–431.

Stoneman, P., and P. Diederen, "Technology Diffusion and Public Policy," *The Economic Journal*, Vol. 104, No. 425, July 1994, pp. 918–930.

Stoneman, P., ed., *Handbook of the Economics of Innovation and Technological Change*, United Kingdom: Blackwell, 1995.

Sultan, F., and L. Chan, "The Adoption of New Technology: The Case of Object-Oriented Computing in Software Companies," *IEEE Transactions on Engineering Management*, Vol. 47, No. 1, 2000, pp. 106–126.

Sultan, F., J. U. Farley, and D. R. Lehmann, "A Meta-Analysis of Applications of Diffusion Models," *Journal of Marketing Research*, Vol. 27, No. 1, 1990, p. 70.

Teng, J.T.C., V. Grover, and W. Guttler, "Information Technology Innovations: General Diffusion Patterns and Its Relationships to Innovation Characteristics," *IEEE Transactions on Engineering Management*, Vol. 49, No. 1, 2002, pp. 13–27.

Tornatzky, L. G., and K. J. Klein, "Innovation Characteristics and Innovation Adoption-Implementation: A Meta-Analysis of Findings," *IEEE Transactions on Engineering Management*, Vol. 29, No. 1, 1982, pp. 28–45.

Tornatzky, L. G., M. Fleischer, et al., *The Processes of Technological Innovation*, Lexington, Mass.: Lexington Books, 1990.

Venkatesh, V., M. Morris, G. Davis, and F. Davis, "User Acceptance of Information Technology: Toward a Unified View," *MIS Quarterly*, Vol. 27, No. 3, 2003, pp. 425–478.

Wang, M., and W. J. Kettinger, "Projecting the Growth of Cellular Communications," *Communications of the Association for Computing Machinery,* Vol. 38, No. 10, 1995, p. 119.

Wolff, E. N., "Productivity, Computerization, and Skill Change," *Economic Review,* Federal Reserve Bank of Atlanta, 2002, pp. 63–87.